Forced Migration and Mental Health

Rethinking the Care of Refugees and Displaced Persons

International and Cultural Psychology Series

Series Editor: **Anthony Marsella**, *University of Hawaii, Honolulu, Hawaii*

A Continuation Order Plan is available for this series. A continuation order will bring delivery of each
new volume immediately upon publication. Volumes are billed only upon actual shipment. For further
information please contact the publisher.

Forced Migration and Mental Health

Rethinking the Care of Refugees and Displaced Persons

Edited by

David Ingleby

Utrecht University
Utrecht, The Netherlands

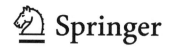 Springer

A C.I.P. Catalogue record for this book is available from the Library of Congress.

ISBN 0-387-22692-3   e-ISBN 0-387-22693-1   Printed on acid-free paper
ISSN 1574-0455

Printed in the United States of America.

9 8 7 6 5 4 3 2 1

springeronline.com

Contributors

Julia Bala is a psychologist and systems-oriented psychotherapist working for Centrum '45 in Amsterdam (Treatment of and research into the consequences of organized violence) and associated with Pharos Foundation (Refugees and Health Knowledge Center) in Utrecht. Educated in former Yugoslavia and the USA, she has a PhD in psychology and her main interests since arriving in the Netherlands in 1992 have been psychotherapy, research and preventive projects related to refugee children and families. She has been developing integrative models for their treatment, intervening on multiple system levels and fostering resilience. She has authored many articles in professional journals and has contributed to several edited volumes.

Ian Clifton-Everest is Senior Lecturer at the Department of Psychology, London Metropolitan University where he teaches Developmental Psychology. He also works in conflict-ridden areas of Africa, South America and the Middle East where he advises on the design of psychosocial programs for the rehabilitation of war-affected children. He has a special interest in the problems of children abducted into fighting forces. He has written on the impact of violence on mental health, on conflict prevention, children's rights, and education for peace and development

Suman Fernando is Honorary Senior Lecturer in Mental Health at the European Centre for Migration and Social Care studies (MASC), University of Kent and Visiting Professor at Department of Applied Social Studies, London Metropolitan University London. He has lectured and written widely on issues of race and culture in mental health. His most recent books are *Mental Health, Race and Culture* (2nd edition Palgrave, 2002) and *Cultural Diversity, Mental Health and Psychiatry. The Struggle against Racism* (Brunner-Routledge, 2003). Suman Fernando is a practicing psychiatrist and is also involved in community organizations providing mental health services to minority ethnic communities in London. He served on the Mental Health Act Commission (a government inspectorate) for nine years until 1995 and chaired its National Standing Committee on Race and Culture.

Choman Hardi does research at the European Centre for Migration and Social Care Studies (MASC), University of Kent. She was born in Kurdistan (Iraq) and during her childhood her family fled twice to Iran. After coming to England in 1993 she studied philosophy and psychology at Queen's College, Oxford and obtained an MA in philosophy at University College, London. She is currently completing her PhD research on the mental health of Kurdish women refugees and has been awarded a Leverhulme Scholarship to study women survivors of Iraq's Anfal campaign against the Kurds.

Choman Hardi is also a writer and has published three collections of poetry in Kurdish and one collection in English (*Life for us*, Bloodaxe Books). She has also facilitated creative writing workshops in the UK and abroad. She was the chair of Exiled Writers' Ink!, an organization of refugee writers.

Anders Hjern is Researcher at the Swedish National Board of Health and Welfare, Centre for Epidemiology, Stockholm and community pediatrician in southern Stockholm. He has a particular interest in public health issues in multicultural societies. He is Associate Professor in Child and Adolescent Medicine at Karolinska Institutet in Stockholm and has published more than 40 articles on public health issues related to inequality and migration in children and youth.

David Ingleby is Professor of Intercultural Psychology at Utrecht University. After working for the Medical Research Council in London and teaching in Social and Political Sciences at Cambridge University, he moved in 1982 to Holland to take up a chair in Developmental Psychology. Since 1991 he has concentrated on issues of migration and culture and was awarded his present chair in 1999. His edited volume *Critical Psychiatry: The politics of mental health* (Pantheon, 1980; Penguin, 1981) has just been reissued by Free Association Books. Together with Charles Watters he teaches in the European MA network on 'Migration, mental health and social care'. He has a lifelong interest in the social dimension of psychology and in interdisciplinary research and practice.

Olle Jeppsson is a Pediatrician at Huddinge University Hospital, Karolinska Institutet, Stockholm. He has been involved with clinical work with refugee families for many years and has also worked on child health in Mozambique, Ethiopia, Angola, Lebanon and Yemen as well as teaching international child health at the Karolinska Institute. During 1993-94 he was employed by Swedish *Save the Children* to evaluate their programme in Kenya for unaccompanied minors from Sudan.

Sander Kramer has been a researcher and teacher at the Utrecht School of Governance, Utrecht University since 1995. He is also a social worker and has experience of residential care and day care for children with learning and developmental problems, as well as prevention programs for migrant youth. His interest in refugees and asylum seekers was broadened by studying Cross-cultural Psychology at Utrecht University. He is currently Course Leader in Utrecht of the European MA on 'Migration, mental health and social care' which is given simultaneously in England, Holland and Sweden.

Derrick Silove is Foundation Professor of Psychiatry at Liverpool Hospital, Sydney (University of New South Wales) and visiting adjunct professor at Karolinska Institutet, Stockholm. He is a long-serving board member of the Service for the Treatment and

Rehabilitation of Torture and Trauma Survivors (STARTTS), Sydney, also working in the Service as a psychiatrist. He currently directs the East Timor National Mental Health Project. His main interest is in pursuing research, advocacy, service planning and social development for refugees, asylum seekers and societies recovering from conflict and oppression. He has published over 150 journal articles, book chapters, monographs and major reports, most in the field of refugee/post-conflict mental health.

Paul Stubbs is Senior Research Fellow, Institute of Economics, Zagreb, Croatia. Born in the UK, he was trained as a sociologist and has lived and worked in Croatia since 1993. He is currently researching the role of international actors in regional development. His main interests, reflected in research, activism and consultancy are: social policy and welfare governance in post-Yugoslav countries; peace-building and social development; community development and mobilization; corporate social responsibility and social reporting; civil society and social movements; online activism; and ethnographies of aid and development. His critical stance on 'war trauma' derives from grassroots work in refugee camps in Croatia and from sociological analyses of mental health professionals. Many of his publications can be downloaded from http://www.gaspp.org (website of the Globalism and Social Policy Programme).

Derek Summerfield is Honorary Senior Lecturer at the Institute of Psychiatry, King's College, London and Research Associate, Refugee Studies Centre, University of Oxford. He was formerly consultant to Oxfam and other aid agencies, and Principal Psychiatrist to the Medical Foundation for Care of Victims of Torture, London. He has been widely involved in training, lecturing and publishing.

Charles Watters is Director of the European Centre for the Study of Migration and Social Care (MASC), University of Kent. He is the author of a number of studies into the mental health and social care of refugees and co-author of a study into good practice in the field, drawing on a range of international examples. Recent interests include research on mental health care for displaced persons in Brazil, an evaluation of the Breathing Space mental health project for refugees, reception arrangements for young refugees in the UK, and comparative international study of pathways to mental health and social care for refugees. He is coordinator of the European MA program 'Migration, mental health and social care'.

Contents

1. EDITOR'S INTRODUCTION

David Ingleby[1]

The phenomenon of forced migration dates back to the beginning of human history. In our time, however, it has become one of the world's major problems. Since 1945 a virtual epidemic of armed conflict, both within and between nations, has created vast numbers of asylum seekers, refugees and displaced persons. This has led in turn to increasing involvement on the part of professional care workers and agencies, both governmental and non-governmental. In the last two decades, the provision of appropriate mental health care for the victims of organized violence has become a major focus of concern.

That care should be provided is - fortunately - increasingly accepted: however, considerable controversy has arisen about the *kind* of care that is necessary. The assumptions and models which initially informed mental health care provision for displaced persons, refugees and asylum seekers have come under scrutiny. As professionals become better acquainted with the problems, alternative approaches are starting to come to the fore.

This book aims to present a critical review of mental health care provisions for these groups of people and to review the controversies currently surrounding this topic. Part I discusses issues arising in humanitarian aid and reconstruction programs; Part II focuses on service provision in host countries. In both areas, we set out to highlight the controversies and new developments.

1. BACKGROUND

In the decades following the end of the Second World War in 1945, the number of armed conflicts in the world increased dramatically. According to the criteria used by Gleditsch et al. (2002), it reached a peak of 56 in 1992, but has been declining since then. This decrease is usually attributed to the ending of the Cold War. Nevertheless, the level of conflict remains alarmingly high and current developments in the Middle East – including the situation in and around Israel and the 'pre-emptive' strike launched against Iraq by a US/UK led coalition in March 2003 – do not bode well for the future.

---

[1] David Ingleby, Faculty of Social Sciences, Utrecht University, The Netherlands

In their survey of global conflict, Marshall and Gurr (2003) have attempted to quantify the total magnitude of armed conflict, taking account not only of the number of conflicts but also their intensity. Figure 1 shows the results of their survey. As can be seen, *internal* conflicts, which typically inflict high levels of suffering on ordinary men, women and children, are by far the most prevalent type of organized violence in the modern world.

Figure 1. The total magnitude of conflict worldwide, as calculated by Marshall (2002)[2]. The uppermost line represents warfare totals; the vertical dashed line indicates the ending of the Cold War in 1991.

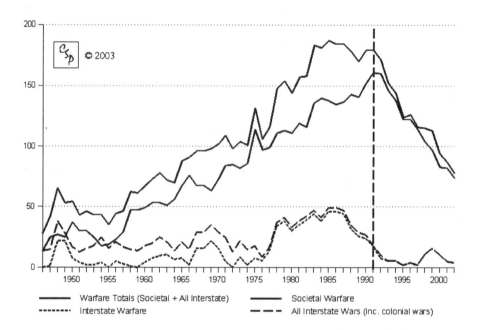

According to the United States Committee for Refugees (USCR)[3], at the end of 2003 some 35.5 million of the world's population had been forced to leave their homes in search of shelter from organized violence. Most of these (23.6 million) remained within the borders of their own country, becoming 'internally displaced persons' (IDP's), while 11.9 million went abroad to become refugees. Figure 2 illustrates the global trends since 1964 in the totals of IDP's and refugees.

---

[2]   Source: CSP (2003). Reproduced by kind permission of the author.
[3]   The statistics quoted here are taken from the *World Refugee Survey 2004* (USCR, 2004). This survey relates to "refugees in need of protection", defined as "asylum seekers awaiting a refugee status determination" plus "refugees who are unwilling or unable to return to their home countries because they fear persecution or armed conflict there and who lack a durable solution".

Figure 2. Totals of displaced persons, 1964-2002[4].

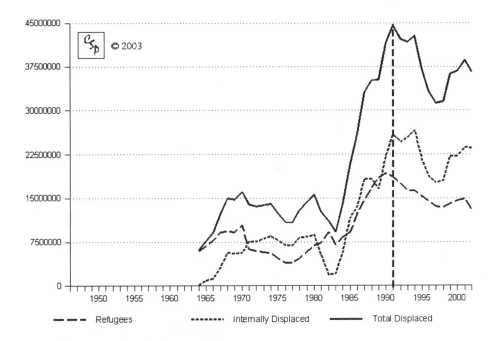

Of course, the amount of forced migration is not simply determined by the level of organized violence. Many other factors play a role. One such factor is transportation – the ease which with migrants can reach another country. Another is government policy, which determines how easy or difficult it is to enter that country and stay in it. Though the 1951 Geneva Convention on Refugees set out to regulate the right to asylum worldwide, differences in the extent to which its provisions have been adopted and in the way they have been implemented have led to wide variations in the accessibility of different countries for those seeking asylum.

At present, the major refugee burden is shouldered by non-Western countries (Middle East 37%, Africa 27% and Southern & Central Asia 16%). Relatively few of those seeking shelter are to be found in European countries (7%), while the combined total for the USA, Canada, Australia and New Zealand is even lower (3%). The 10% who flee to the West are almost by definition a select and atypical group, able to plan, pay for and undertake a hazardous and uncertain enterprise.

---

[4] Source: CSP (2003). Reproduced by kind permission of the author. Data derived from the USCR's *World Refugee Surveys.*

Since the 1970s the proportion of refugees reaching Western countries has increased considerably, mainly because of better transport facilities. However, the surge which industrialized countries experienced during the 1990s had a political backlash: it led to a tightening-up of the laws and procedures governing asylum which is still going on. Together with the decline in the amount of conflict world-wide, this has led in the last three years to a fall in the annual numbers of those seeking asylum in Western countries (see Figure 3), as well as the proportion who are allowed to stay.

Figure 3. Annual asylum applications in 36 industrialized countries, 1980–2003[5].

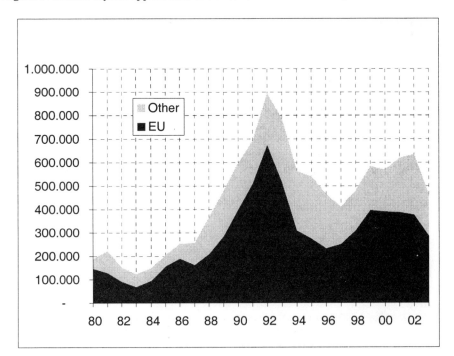

As can be seen, asylum applications in industrialized countries increased nearly ten-fold between 1983 and the peak year 1992. Subsequently, the number of asylum seekers declined – partly due to the ending of certain conflicts, but also to the adoption of the increasingly stringent policies referred to above. Towards the end of the 1990s, the figures rose again, but in the last three years they have shown a steady decrease: 614,650 in 2001, 579,040 in 2002 and 463,130 in 2003.

In a relative sense, then, the pressure is off Western governments concerned about a 'tidal wave' of asylum seekers 'swamping' their countries – at least for the time being. However, these statistics can be misleading. They say nothing about the numbers of forced migrants entering countries illegally, or the number of asylum seekers who disappear into illegality after their application is rejected. As policies in Western

---

[5] Source: UNHCR (2004), p. 4. Reproduced by kind permission of the Population Data Unit, UNHCR Geneva.

countries have become stricter, the numbers of these 'undocumented' migrants have increased – though since these are people who officially do not exist, it is of course hard to obtain reliable estimates. Anders Hjern and Olle Jeppsson draw attention to this increasing human rights problem in Chapter 7.

Moreover, the recent decline in the number of asylum applications in industrialized countries does not make the problem of providing adequate care any less urgent. This problem does not concern only the newcomers, but also those who may already have spent several years in the host country.

2. PHASES IN THE DEVELOPMENT OF SERVICE PROVISION

The provision of effective health and social care for asylum seekers and refugees is partly motivated by principles of human rights and partly by pragmatic considerations. The right to care is laid down in the 1951 Geneva Convention on Refugees; more recently, the European Commission adopted on 27th January 2003 a directive laying down minimum standards on the reception of asylum applicants in Member States, including standards of health care. But apart from the question of human rights, governments also have an interest in ensuring that this group is not neglected. Ignoring the problems people have usually leads to more serious problems at a later stage. For example, a refugee handicapped by psychosocial problems is likely to have difficulty getting a job and integrating into the host society, thereby becoming even more dependent on the state.

2.1. Prior to 1980

In the period preceding the dramatic rise in the number of refugees during the 1980s, the concept of humanitarian aid was restricted to the provision of the most basic necessities: food, water, shelter and basic medical care. These were the priorities of the relief programs organized by NGO's working with IDP's and with refugees in the countries surrounding a conflict zone. In a sense, these remain the priorities for relief programs in any setting, because it is universally recognized that basic material needs have to be met before psychological and social problems can be properly dealt with.

However, for refugees who had sought refuge in Western countries, psychological help was also available. Once admitted to a country, refugees could make use of its mental health services. The numbers concerned were small and there are few data on the demand for services and their adequacy. Nevertheless, it is clear that one category of problems received special attention: physical and psychological disorders resulting from torture or exposure to other forms of violence. Treatment for these problems was often provided by professionals with prior experience in helping victims of the Second World War and other armed conflicts. This is the background of centers such as the Medical Foundation for the Care of Victims of Torture (Britain) or Icodo and Centrum '45 (The Netherlands). Insofar as there was special provision for refugees in this period, we can say that the mental health services viewed refugees primarily as *victims of organized violence*.

2.2. The 1980s

From about 1980 onwards we see a dramatic increase in the attention paid to the psychological problems of refugees, accompanying a steep rise in their numbers. One rough-and-ready way of quantifying this attention is by examining the number of articles published in the scientific literature which make reference to refugees. If we do this for the medical literature, using the MEDLINE database, we can see a small but steady interest in refugees from 1968 to 1977, which then increases dramatically until 1995, falling back slightly after that date. The psychological literature can be surveyed in the same way using the PsycINFO database: this shows the same general pattern, but the expansion between 1977 and 1995 is much more marked. In the last two decades, therefore, we see that psychological attention for refugee problems has increased faster than medical attention.

In absolute terms, there are many more medical publications than psychological ones, but even in these terms the trend is clear. Between 1968 and 1982 there were seven medical articles mentioning refugees for every psychological article. After 1982, however, this ratio was only about 2:1. Figure 4 shows the rise in the percentage of publications mentioning refugees in both areas.

Figure 4. Percentage of all publications in the medical and psychological literature in which the words 'refugee' or 'refugees' appear in the bibliographical data (title, summary, keywords)[6]. The year 1970 stands for the period 1968–1972, 1975 for 1973–1978, etc.

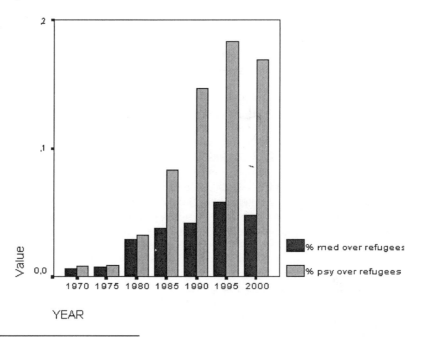

---

[6] Source of data for figures 4-6: Ovid Technologies ERL® WebSPIRS® 5.

When we examine the *content* of the psychological articles concerned with refugees, we see that they continue to be primarily focused on the effects of past sufferings: there is little attention to the effects of forced migration itself or the problems of readjustment in a new country. In the field, psychosocial teams began to be sent to conflict regions by NGO's during the 1980s to work alongside those providing material relief and basic medical care. This increased activity owed a great deal to the sudden upswing in the acceptance of the concept of 'trauma'.

Most commentators agree that the origin of the new concern for traumatization lay in the Vietnam War. Many U.S. conscripts returned home with psychological problems and difficulties of adjustment, but the military authorities at first denied any link between these problems and their war experiences. Acceptance of the concept of 'post-traumatic stress disorder' as a psychiatric category was signaled in 1980 by its adoption in the Diagnostic and Statistical Manual of the American Psychiatric Association. This was a victory for groups lobbying for the interests of Vietnam veterans. It entitled veterans to the treatment, the public sympathy and the financial assistance which up until then they had mostly been denied. The diagnosis of PTSD, in the words of Summerfield (2001), "was meant to shift the focus of attention from the details of a soldier's background and psyche to the fundamentally traumatogenic nature of war". The current diagnostic criteria for PTSD include a specification of the traumatizing event (actual or threatened death or serious injury, etc.) and the patient's response to it (intense fear, helpless, horror etc.), together with the three characteristic symptoms:

1. Persistent *re-experiencing* of the traumatic event (distressing images, night-mares, flashbacks etc.), causing distress and signs of panic;
2. Persistent *avoidance* of stimuli associated with the trauma, numbing of general responsiveness.
3. Persistent symptoms of increased *arousal* (e.g. insomnia, irritability, concentration problems, hypervigilance and increased startle responses).

All these symptoms must be present and severe enough to cause substantial impairment in social, occupational or interpersonal domains. Moreover, the symptoms must be present for at least one month.

2.3. The explosive growth of the trauma approach

Originally developed in the light of the experiences of Vietnam veterans, the PTSD concept also became widely used in relation to victims of sexual and domestic violence, accidents and natural disasters, as well as organized violence. The notion of 'having a trauma' became part of everyday language. Trauma therapy became a flourishing specialty, most treatments being based on some version of the notion of 'working through' or re-experiencing of the traumatizing events. Quite apart from the relief these treatments brought, the diagnosis of PTSD offered victims of violence the possibility of social recognition and financial compensation.

Some idea of the spectacular increase in the amount of attention paid to trauma can be obtained from Figure 5, which shows the percentage of publications during successive 5-year periods in which the concepts 'trauma', 'psychotrauma' or 'PTSD' figure in the PsycINF database. It is worth noting that publications over refugees make up only a tiny fraction of the trauma literature: during the past 15 years this proportion has remained steady at around 3%.

Figure 5. Percentage of publications in the psychological literature with the words 'trauma', 'psychotrauma' or 'PTSD' in the bibliographical data.

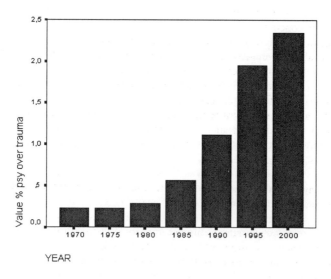

Figure 6. Percentage of articles in PsycINF with the words 'refugee' or 'refugees', in combination with the words 'trauma', 'psychotrauma' or 'PTSD', in the bibliographical data.

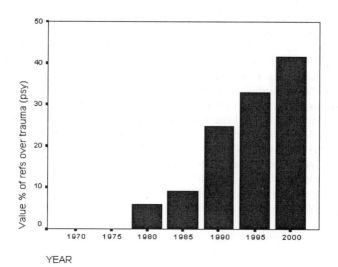

The way in which the trauma concept suddenly rose to prominence has attracted much attention as a social phenomenon in its own right. Notions of 'medicalization', 'social construction' and 'professional imperialism' were applied to this phenomenon by authors whom we will discuss in later sections. The extent to which the trauma concept came to dominate the psychological study of refugees can be seen very clearly in Figure 6, which shows the percentage of articles on refugees in which the concept figures. Whereas there are *no* mentions of 'trauma' in connection with refugees during the decade 1968-1977, almost half of all psychological articles on refugees during the last five years make reference to the concept.

A simple statistical analysis enables us to answer the following question: is the number of publications about "refugees and trauma" primarily related to the level of interest in refugees, or to the level of interest in trauma? Multiple regression analysis reveals the existence of a highly significant relationship with the latter variable, yet none at all with the former. This is an extremely interesting finding: it suggests that it was trauma researchers who became interested in refugees, rather than refugee researchers becoming interested in trauma. More detailed analysis of the literature would be necessary to confirm this interpretation, but it suggests that the research in this field has been more 'theory-driven' than 'problem-driven'.

From about 1980 onwards, then, the concept of 'trauma' increasingly formed the basis of studies and interventions concerning the mental health needs of refugees, whether they were living in the industrialized West or in conflict zones. Very soon, the trauma approach became a self-perpetuating, almost closed system. Criticism of the one-sidedness of this approach was routinely waved aside as callous indifference to the plight of those suffering. The word 'trauma' itself was used to describe *both* the situation causing the disturbance, *and* the disturbance itself: this elision reinforced the notion that if a situation was 'traumatic', those experiencing it would automatically be 'traumatized'. Yet many studies show large, unexplained variations in the extent to which experiences of violence lead to symptoms of PTSD.

In many studies, only data related to PTSD were collected: other ways of looking at refugees' problems were not considered. Data were routinely collected using diagnostic instruments which had never been validated for the population studied. A recent example of this was a study in Sierra Leone (De Jong et al., 2000) which reported that 99% of respondents had scores on the Impact of Events Scale (IES) "that indicated very high levels of disturbances, indicative of severe PTSD in western Europe". Although the first author later modified this claim (De Jong, 2001), it is entirely typical of the tendency to 'talk up the numbers' which characterized, for example, reports by NGO's during the Balkans Wars (see Paul Stubbs in Chapter 3).

Some authors ascribe traumas to whole populations, giving the concept an extremely broad interpretation which bears little relation to the official definition of PTSD. An example of this can be seen in a report on the children of Iraq, undertaken in the run-up to the invasion in 2003 (International Study Team, 2003, p. 6): "Iraqi children are already badly traumatized by 12 years of economic sanctions". Some people evidently feel that the end justifies the means, as long as such statements generate more concern for victims of violence: but perhaps refugees and asylum seekers would be better served by more respect for the precise nature of their problems.

2.4. Growing doubts about PTSD

During the 1990's, as we can see from Figures 5 and 6, the popularity of the 'trauma' approach continued to increase. Nevertheless – almost inevitably, when we consider how uncritically the trauma approach was embraced to begin with – doubts soon began to be voiced about the universality and relevance of the PTSD diagnosis. Kleber et al. (1995) and Marsella et al. (1996) marshal some of these criticisms.

- Authors such as Kleber et al. (1992) argued for toning down the pathological connotations of PTSD by introducing a distinction between 'normal' and 'abnormal' ways of reacting to extreme stress: the former was designated as 'Post Traumatic Stress *Reaction*'. (This view receives support from a recent article by Yehuda (2003), which argues that 're-experiencing', 'avoidance' and 'arousal' are virtually universal reactions to extremely shocking experiences, and that PTSD should be seen as the *abnormal persistence* of these symptoms.)

- The DSM definition of 'trauma' presupposes one or more catastrophic events, capable of being localized in space and time. This, however, does not do justice to the fact that refugees have often experienced a long series of stressful events. The concept of 'sequential traumatization', developed by the Dutch psychiatrist Keilson in the course of his work with child survivors of the holocaust (Keilson & Sarphati, 1979) struck many critics as more appropriate.

- Researchers such as Silove (1999) pointed out that the prevalence of PTSD among refugees was highly variable and that it is hard to predict, purely on the basis of what someone has experienced, whether they will develop the condition. Kessler et al. (1995) had already noted that only 9% of men and 20% of women who were exposed to a potentially traumatizing experience in terms of the DSM criteria, actually developed symptoms of the disorder.

- Others (e.g. Summerfield, 1999) regarded the emphasis on PTSD as misplaced. People with PTSD symptoms may not regard them as their most serious problem, and such symptoms may not always cause much impairment of functioning. Chapter 4 by Olle Jeppsson and Anders Hjern, a study of the 'lost boys of Sudan', provides a graphic example of this. In an epidemiological study of 824 asylum seekers from Kosovo in Great Britain (Summerfield, 2002), almost all respondents mentioned *work, schooling* and *family reunification* as their major concerns; very few respondents seemed to be bothered by their psychological symptoms. This finding contrasts sharply with the conclusions of Turner et al. (2003), who studied the same group of 824 asylum seekers and estimated that half of them had PTSD.

- A number of authors (e.g. Summerfield, 1999, Angel et al., 2001) have expressed doubts about the advisability of therapies involving 'working through' for people whose cultures place a high value on stoicism and 'active forgetting'.

Alongside these specific points of criticism, the limitations of the PTSD concept led to many frustrations among refugee mental health workers and their clients. Like a narrow funnel, the concept seemed to reduce both *causes* and *effects* to a drastically simplified form, which on its own was seldom encountered in practice – at any rate among refugees. This led to a sort of 'tunnel vision' among mental health workers, researchers, policy makers and financial donors, in which awareness of other problems was seriously attenuated.

- The *causes* of the psychological problems of refugees cannot be reduced to a single catastrophic, life-threatening event, or even to a sequence of such events. Not knowing what the fate of one's family is, for example, or whether one will obtain asylum, is not an *event* but a *situation*. There is a further difference between a refugee and the accidental victim of a plane crash or an armed robbery. The traumatic events which refugees have experienced do not come out of the blue, but are intimately connected with the rest of their lives. They are embedded in a context of threat, uncertainty, deprivation, oppression and suffering. As Shakespeare put it *(Hamlet, Act iv. sc. 5)*: "when sorrows come, they come not single spies, but in battalions". The concept of PTSD thus focuses on only a part of the stressful experiences which most refugees have undergone.

- Likewise, the PTSD concept focuses on a small selection of the *effects* of these experiences. Out of the whole panoply of forms of psychological (and other) problems which this group can suffer from, three symptoms are singled out: re-experiencing, avoidance and arousal. Anything which does not fall under these headings is relegated to the category of 'co-morbidity'. This hardly does justice to the wide range of complaints which those working with refugees encounter daily. Considered from the perspective of system theory (see Chapter 10 by Julia Bala), the PTSD diagnosis is even more inadequate, because the concept refers only to the individual patient and does not consider possible disturbances of the social system in which they operate. Some problems may go beyond the boundaries of what is usually designated 'mental health': consider, for example the *moral* crisis which Ian Clifton-Everest describes (Chapter 5) in former child soldiers. In sum, PTSD focuses attention on a highly limited cluster of symptoms, which may cause great hardship to some refugees, but may be totally absent among others, or overshadowed by more complex problems.

Even though the 1990s saw the emergence of critical views on PTSD, the concept continued to dominate the field of mental health care for refugees. However, other approaches began to receive attention. Other disciplines started paying more attention to the problems of refugees – in particular, anthropology, where publications on this topic showed a marked upturn in the 1990s. As a result, other issues apart from 'trauma' were introduced, problematizing the situation of refugees in different ways. In this way, the field of refugee mental health care has recently become an unusually lively and controversial scientific arena, with a wealth of different viewpoints competing for attention. In the following section we will identify some of the different perspectives which have influenced thinking about service provision.

3. SCHOOLS OF THOUGHT INFLUENCING SERVICE PROVISION

Watters (2001) has presented a review of 'emerging paradigms' in the care for refugees; the following discussion overlaps to some extent with that article. It should be borne in mind that the 'schools' we discuss are 'ideal types'. It is often unclear where the boundaries between schools lie and who the main protagonists are: on some issues, different schools may overlap with each other. As a starting-point, however, we propose the following rough taxonomy.

1. Mainstream health care approaches
2. Multicultural mental health care
3. Sociological approaches
4. 'Managed care'
5. The role of users' movements.

3.1. Mainstream health care approaches

It is a mistake to assume that 'mainstream' health care represents a uniform way of thinking. Quite apart from 'alternative' medicine, there is a broad spectrum of established approaches. One way of ordering these is on a continuum from 'hard' (positivistic) approaches to 'soft' (humanistic or interpretative) ones.

At the 'hard' end of the spectrum is the biomedical model, embraced by psychiatrists, neurologists and clinical psychologists who attempt to model their work on the natural sciences. Within the field of mental health, this approach came under heavy fire from the critics of the 1960s and 1970s, but since then it has made a remarkable comeback. This approach pays scant attention to the social context and meaning of people's complaints; symptoms are described as 'objectively' as possible and successful treatment is equated with their removal. The symptoms, one might say, are the target of attention – not the person who is bothered by them. (In clinical medicine, indeed, it is still commonplace to talk about 'the brain tumor in bed three').

What we refer to as 'soft' approaches to health care are those in which a more important role is accorded to the social context and meaning of behavior and experience. The most important are perhaps *psychotherapeutic* approaches, the classical exponents of which are such figures as Sigmund Freud and Carl Rogers, and *social medicine* and *public health* approaches.

3.1.1. Positivist, biomedical approaches

In these approaches, refugees' problems are most often described in terms of PTSD, seen as a specific psychiatric disorder and formulated in terms conforming to the biomedical paradigm and the 'descriptive' nosological tradition of Emil Kraepelin. For Kraepelin, mental disorders were illnesses like any others: the advancement of medical science required a precise, objective description of the symptoms of the illness, in which the meaning, context and suspected cause of the symptoms played as small a role as possible. Workers in the psychodynamic tradition, in particular, have looked on in dismay as present-day Kraepelinians have gained more and more influence within the mental health field – particularly during recent revisions of the DSM (the Diagnostic and

Statistical Manual of the American Psychiatric Association). Since the DSM forms the basis of mental health practice in many Western countries, this represents a substantial shift of power.

In one conspicuous respect, however, as Young (2002) has pointed out, PTSD does *not* fit into a purely descriptive approach to nosology: the supposed cause is part of the definition, constituting one of the *criteria* for the disorder. In all other respects, however, the concept fits perfectly into the biomedical tradition. Nevertheless, this tradition is only one of many which are represented in the whole field of mental health. Mental health care is not a homogenous entity, but a complex arena in which different disciplines, professions and approaches continually struggle for supremacy. The debates which have arisen about PTSD, therefore, are anything but unexpected: they reflect fundamental and persistent tensions within health care itself.

3.1.2. Psychotherapeutic approaches

Here – in contrast – the experience of the client occupies a central place and 'idiographic' (one-off) characterizations are preferred to standardized diagnostic instruments. Compared to the Kraepelinian approach, much more attention is paid to the relational context of the individual. Moreover, the client's general well-being and level of functioning is regarded as more important than merely the presence or absence of symptoms. The task of the therapist is seen in terms of communicating, conferring and negotiating with the client, rather than as applying a 'treatment' in the medical sense. The psychotherapeutic approach can also be characterized as a 'humanistic' one, because the client is seen as an *agent* and a *subject* rather than a passive 'patient', wholly at the mercy of external forces. Another important difference is that while the biomedical approach focuses on 'disease', psychotherapeutic approaches attend to 'illness' (see section 3.2 for a discussion of this contrast).

3.1.3. The social medicine or public health tradition

This approach differs from the biomedical one in two respects. Firstly, more attention is paid to peoples' social and physical environment: social medicine focuses both on a person's place in society, and on the place of illness in their life. Secondly, social medicine is not simply concerned with symptom reduction, but also with the promotion of health. Moreover, health – according to the famous definition written into the constitution of the World Health Organization in 1948 – is seen as "a state of complete physical, mental, and social well-being and not merely the absence of disease or infirmity". According to this view, health care is not only concerned with pathology, but with the whole range of conditions (including the social context) which influence health in this broad sense.

Exponents of the social medicine or public health tradition have played an important role in shaping the identity of the WHO and – at both national and international levels – in setting up policies concerned with the care of refugees. In the Netherlands, for example, the centre which the Government set up to coordinate health care for refugees (Pharos) worked from this perspective and the publications of its first director, Loes van Willigen, provide a good illustration of its scientific principles (see, e.g., Van Willigen & Hondius, 1992; Van Willigen (ed.), 2000; Van Willigen, 2003). In mental health care, this approach is closely related to the 'mental hygiene movement' which played a vital role during the twentieth century in developing alternatives to the biomedical model. It is an approach which regards *prevention* as no less important than *cure,* paying detailed attention to the sources of stress and disability which may be located in the present environment of refugees and asylum seekers. Such an emphasis is more often found in the field of *primary care* than among providers of specialized, clinical services. In the present volume, Chapter 7 by Anders Hjern and Olle Jeppsson provides a good example of work in the tradition of social medicine and public health.

Closely related to this tradition are the so-called 'psychosocial' approaches to the care of refugees, which are often underlie reconstruction work in post-conflict societies. Chapter 2 by Derrick Silove and Chapter 3 by Paul Stubbs devote specific attention to these approaches. Silove also gives prominence to a third approach, which he calls the 'severe mental illness' model. This approach focuses on a group which is relatively small in size (1% or more), but urgently in need of help because of severe emotional or behavioral disorders. Some of these individuals may have been disturbed before the conflict situation arose; whatever the cause of their problems, Silove argues that the excessive focus of debate on the trauma model has diverted attention from their needs.

3.1.4. Observations on theoretical approaches to refugee mental health care

When we examine the competing paradigms within the field of mental health, we see that the criticisms of PTSD listed above are not simply directed at the concept itself, but at the positivistic model of clinical practice which gave rise to the concept of PTSD in the first place.

I have referred above to the criticism of PTSD as a 'funnel' that narrows down both causes and effects to a stripped-down version (a criticism that has often been voiced by workers in the psychotherapeutic and public health traditions). The great riddle of PTSD is this: how did a concept that is so incapable of doing justice to the experience of mental health workers and their clients come to occupy a position of exclusive dominance in the field of mental health care for refugees? Are the proponents of PTSD really so powerful and cunning, and the professionals and their clients so naïve, that almost everyone failed to notice the glaring inadequacy of the concept?

In section 3.3 I will suggest that the emphasis on PTSD can only be understood if we consider the *social consequences* of such a diagnosis. Similar paradoxes can be found in other areas of health care. Certain concepts drawn from the biomedical tradition, for example 'anorexia nervosa' or 'attention deficit hyperactivity disorder' (ADHD), are applied far more often than is strictly warranted in terms of the clinical criteria. Yet the popularity of these labels is easier to understand when we take account of the sociological dimensions of sickness, in particular the question of power: sometimes a biomedical category has to be used *in order to get things done.* Before developing this point further, however, I will first examine other approaches which have been applied in research and care programs for refugees.

3.1.5. Eclecticism

What is immediately striking when surveying this area is the enormous diversity of both the theories and methods adopted, and the problems to which they are applied. Despite the dominance of the PTSD concept, alongside the purely 'clinical' approach there is ample attention for the context of the refugees' lives and the myriad factors which can influence their well-being. This diversity of approaches is not surprising when we consider the diverse sorts of professionals in collaboration with whom this theoretical knowledge has been generated: not only clinicians but also general practitioners, youth workers, teachers, voluntary workers and policy makers.

Theory development in this area has thus a predominately *eclectic* character. Even clinicians concerned explicitly with the treatment of 'trauma' seldom limit themselves to a symptom-oriented, Kraepelinian approach: most of them also try to pay attention to 'the person in context'. True, some therapies (for example, 're-exposure therapies' such as 'implosion' or 'flooding') are narrowly focused on the symptoms of PTSD. But most therapies used for trauma patients have a much broader focus: indeed, there is hardly any form of therapy which has *not* been applied to this group! This fact is not as strange as it sounds, when we take account of the fact that PTSD can be accompanied by depression, anxiety, addiction, relation problems, aggressive disorders and even schizophrenia. Nevertheless, when the client is a refugee, it is usually the PTSD symptoms which are highlighted: the rest tends to be seen as merely 'co-morbidity'.

3.1.6. Prevention

Another important theme in research and theory development in this area is *prevention*. Especially in the so-called 'psycho-social' approach, models of normal functioning such as Garmezy's (1985) model of 'risk factors' and 'protective factors' are applied to the question of fostering the well-being of refugees. Also popular in this field is the 'stress and coping' model of Lazarus and Folkman (1984).

Occasionally, a concern with prevention leads mental health workers to become involved in advocacy or political campaigns for the dignity and human rights of refugees and asylum seekers. 'Professional detachment' has nothing to do with turning a blind eye to social wrongs, and health care workers are sometimes the only witnesses to these wrongs. In such cases, their duty is not only to help their patients, but to ensure that the injustices that they have witnessed are dealt with. Those concerned with the care of refugees and asylum seekers are constantly confronted with examples of disregard for the human rights of this vulnerable group. Many refugees who have fled to neighboring countries are victims of what the U.S. Committee for Refugees (op. cit.) has dubbed 'warehousing': more than 7 million of the world's 12 million refugees have been confined for ten years or more in camps or separate settlements. This disregard is also manifested in the way in which asylum seekers are treated in prosperous Western countries by lawmakers, bureaucrats, state organizations, media and the general public. Lately, human rights organizations have expressed particular concern about the detention policies operated by (among others) the UK, Australia and the USA, and the deportation policy for those refused asylum – sometimes after years spent living in the host country – by the Netherlands. 'Group advocacy' and public protest against these forms of injustice is an integral part of the care worker's responsibility (see Silove et al., 2000; Ingleby, 2001).

The problem with effective care delivery for refugees and asylum seekers, as will become clear in the following chapters, has nothing to do with a shortage of theoretical perspectives and research findings on this topic. On the contrary, a wealth of ideas and research is available, and the problems of refugees have been approached from many angles. The problem of providing care for this group, as Ingleby and Watters argue in Chapter 12, is to *integrate* all these different perspectives – to provide 'holistic' care in which all the different problems refugees can have are tackled in a coherent way, rather than being divided up between services that are more inclined to compete with each other than to cooperate.

3.2. Multicultural mental health care

As Suman Fernando points out in Chapter 11, the care of refugees is almost always *multicultural* care. In the last two decades there has been an upsurge of interest in the relevance of the cultural context to all types of service provision.

In the 1950s the discipline of 'transcultural psychiatry' came into being. This branch of psychiatry is concerned both with service provision in different countries and with problems within culturally or ethnically diverse societies. The effects of migration and the problems of migrants are a central topic in this branch of health care. During the 1990s we see steadily more focus on *the refugee as migrant,* supplementing and sometimes replacing the emphasis on *the refugee as victim of organized violence.* Within this approach, the problems of service provision for refugees are viewed in relation to multicultural service provision in general. This has encouraged concern for the other kinds of problems refugees may have apart from traumatic experiences in the past.

3.2.1. Refugees as migrants

An important article marking the shift towards viewing the refugee as a migrant was published by Van Dijk (1996). This shift occurred during a decade in which refugees were beginning to make up a significant proportion of the migrant population. Up to the mid-1980s, the numbers of refugees were very small and care for them was mostly pro-vided outside the mainstream. There was little common ground between professionals and services dealing with refugees and those helping other immigrants. Refugee clients were often well educated and were regarded as having a rather esoteric clinical problem (trauma), calling for specialized individual psychotherapy. At least until the late 1980s, the public image of the refugee was also generally positive: refugees enjoyed a sort of moral credit, in the eyes of the public, which labor migrants totally lacked. This gave them an almost self-evident right to respect, compassion and help.

Professionals helping labor migrants, on the other hand, mostly had clients with low educational qualifications and low incomes, who displayed a range of diffuse and over-lapping problems often related to a socially marginal or disadvantaged position. Psycho-therapy was seldom felt to be suitable for these clients, who were often shunted directly into intramural care or social psychiatry. For a variety of reasons, then, there was little overlap and exchange of views between those working with refugees and those concerned with multicultural health care in general.

Within health and social care, however, the contrast between 'political' and 'labor' migrants is beginning to blur. Firstly, the dominant public image of asylum seekers has changed. Far from being moral heroes, they are often viewed nowadays as moral black-mailers, exploiting the goodwill of the host nation to gain access in a fraudulent way to welfare benefits. This may be a question of political attitudes, but in certain ways the reality has also changed. In recent years, an increasing proportion of asylum seekers with low educational qualifications have migrated to the West from non-industrialized countries. Moreover, it has become obvious that the problems of refugees and asylum seekers are not confined to PTSD, but also concern less esoteric problems such as aggression, school maladjustment, family conflicts and drug or alcohol addiction - the roots of which are just as likely to be found in the present situation as in the past. So we see that it is not only the *profile* of asylum seekers that has moved closer to that of other immigrants; so too have their *problems*.

Added to this, there has been a recent shift towards integrating services for refugees within regular health and social care provisions. In the UK, this has been a consequence of the new policy of 'dispersing' refugees in remote areas of the country. Regions such as Northumberland – parts of which have seen few foreigners since the Roman soldiers who built Hadrian's Wall – suddenly found themselves having to provide health and social care to new arrivals from all over the globe. In the Netherlands, a dispersal policy had been in place since the 1980s, though up until 2000 most care was provided within accommodation centers. After that date, these separate services were scaled down and asylum seekers had to make use of 'mainstream' facilities. In both countries, the integra-tion of refugee services into regular health care has given a new impetus to the development of multicultural care provisions.

The sheer numerical increase in the proportion of refugees in the population is another factor working against separate service provision. In Western countries, particu-larly those with a highly restrictive policy on labor immigration, refugees make up a considerable proportion of the immigrant population. The result of all these developments has been to bring those concerned with the care of refugees in closer contact with those developing care services for a culturally diverse population.

3.2.2. The evolution of multicultural mental health care

The cross-cultural study of psychiatric conditions begins in the colonial era with studies by psychiatrists and anthropologists of the disorders found among 'natives' or 'aboriginals'. The description of these disorders was strongly biased by assumptions about white supremacy; writers tended to produce descriptions which emphasized the 'otherness' of the colonized peoples and the 'exotic' or 'bizarre' nature of their distur-bances. The study of 'culture-bound' disorders has its roots in this period.

One nineteenth-century psychiatrist who broke with this tradition was Emil Kraepelin, regarded by many as 'the father of modern psychiatry'. His classic work on transcultural psychiatry (Kraepelin, 1904) was the result of an expedition to Java to validate the concepts of dementia praecox and manic depression. Instead of stressing the 'otherness' of the native, Kraepelin was concerned with the opposite: to demonstrate the universal applicability of his biologically based classification system. However, his pioneering work was not continued until half a century later.

The development of modern 'transcultural psychiatry' received a boost from the founding of the WHO, which initiated the first systematic attempts to study health on a worldwide basis and to coordinate global health policy. This work had a firmly universalistic starting-point. Western disease categories and Western treatment methods were assumed to be relevant in all countries; at most, a little 'fine tuning' would be required to adapt them to different cultural settings. The provision of 'culturally sensitive care' was seen, at most, as a question of accurately translating universal core concepts of illness and treatment into different cultural idioms.

In service provision within multicultural societies during and after the 1950s, the same assumption can be discerned: the basis of service provision was the model developed within the (white) majority culture. Immigrants were expected to adapt whatever notions about sickness and health they might have on arrival to conform to this model. In this respect, health policy was in line with the 'assimilationist' approach to migration in this period.

However, from the 1970s onwards a shift away from universalistic, Western-centered approaches to a more relativistic version of transcultural psychiatry can be discerned. On the global level, Kleinman (1988) criticized the epidemiological studies of the WHO and promoted the discipline of 'anthropological psychiatry'. In the major Western nations, the shift from 'monocultural' to 'multicultural' social policies was reflected in increasing concern for 'culturally appropriate' service provision. This was a logical consequence of the notion of equal rights and citizenship for members of all ethnic groups. It was not enough to ensure that all groups were offered the same care, because *identical* care for minorities actually meant *inadequate* care. Thus, from around 1980 we see major efforts to improve the accessibility and quality of care provisions for minority groups. Similar efforts were undertaken in the field of education.

3.2.3. Principles of multicultural care

Central to modern multicultural health care is the distinction between 'disease' and 'illness'. According to Kleinman (1981, p. 72), "disease refers to a malfunctioning of biological and/or psychological processes, while the term illness refers to the psychosocial experience and meaning of perceived disease". Whereas it is possible that certain disease processes have universal characteristics, *illness* in the sense described above is inextricably linked with its social and cultural context. Cultural factors do not simply affect the superficial appearance ('presentation') of psychological disorders: they influence their genesis, recognition, course and remedy.

According to this view, multicultural health care is not simply a matter of formulating Western categories and treatments in the appropriate local idioms. Problems are inevitably shaped by the framework of social meanings which structures thought and feeling. Moreover, the *social* consequences of having a particular illness can influence its course drastically. Thus, culture plays a role at all stages of an illness: in its causation, the way it is construed and experienced, the accessibility of treatment, the response of the professional, the form of treatment given and its effectiveness, and the prognosis for later life.

Such an approach is hard to reconcile with the standard procedures of Western mental health care, which pay little attention to the social context of illness and its treatment. In the biomedical model, the individual is regarded in isolation from his or her cultural, political, economic and historical context. Trauma, loss, grief, mourning, break-down, coping, healing and recovery are all regarded in current clinical models as *intra-psychic* processes, whereas the reality is that they are embedded in a cultural and social context. They are things that people go through *together* - not simply in 'collectivist' non-Western cultures, but the world over. A steadily increasingly number of anthropological studies (see, for example, Summerfield, 1995; Robben & Suárez-Oroczo, 2000) has shown how indispensable an anthropological approach is in understanding the supposedly intrapsychic processes that clinicians refer to.

Important for the quality of service delivery, and thus to the definition of 'good practice', is the 'goodness of fit' or 'matching' between the help offered and the people receiving it. Help must *make sense* to the recipients and take account of their life-style and current situation. Kleinman et al. (1978) used the term 'explanatory models' to describe people's ideas concerning their illness (its cause, timing, effects, mechanism, severity, duration, prognosis), the kind of treatment they thought appropriate, and their hopes and fears. This concept has played a seminal role in work aimed at 'matching' service provision to users.

For multicultural health care, the life world and meaning systems of users must become important objects of study. Moreover, such study must consist of more than fill-ing in predetermined response categories in standardized questionnaires: it must use *qualitative* methods which give a voice to the persons studied and allow them to answer within their own perspective (cf. Chapter 8). To carry this approach to its logical conclusion, users themselves must play a role in designing services. Both in research and policy-making, the 'new transcultural psychiatry' (Littlewood, 1990) implies a radical shift in the balance of power away from researchers and professionals and towards users: a 'bottom-up' instead of 'top-down' approach. This gives a much more radical meaning to the notion of 'cultural sensitivity'. Instead of being seen purely as a matter of bridging a communication gap, this notion actually implies *changing the culture of service providers themselves*.

3.2.4. Rethinking the concept of 'culture'

From about 1995 onwards, new developments have occurred in the field of multi-cultural care which challenge the notion of 'culture' previously assumed by transcultural psychiatrists. These developments are related to emerging views within anthropology. Firstly, Geertz (1973) argued replacement of the static, monolithic concept of 'culture' with an approach that does justice to the heterogeneous and dynamic nature of real cultures. Instead of treating culture as a categorical variable on which each individual can be assigned a single value, we should recognize that many people position themselves simultaneously within two or more cultures: this is especially true for migrants. Secondly, researchers on ethnicity influenced by Barth (1969) have argued that 'culture' itself has no objective existence, but should be viewed as a social construction: cultural properties are actually 'ethnic markers', called into being when strategic considerations make them necessary. The example of Bosnia-Herzegovina is sometimes cited - a society in which cultural differences were allegedly not regarded as important until the outbreak of war between ethnic groups in 1992.

In retrospect, then, early attempts to put culture on the agenda of health care may have led us down a blind alley. 'Cultural sensitivity' has often been often interpreted as adapting service delivery to the cultural peculiarities of different racial or ethnic groups (Blacks, Hispanics, Asians, Moroccans, etc.). Yet whether these groups actually exist as culturally homogeneous categories is highly questionable; the effect of using these distinctions may have merely been to reinforce existing myths and stereotypes and actually *increase* the distance between service providers and users.

Treating cultural differences as objective phenomena forming inevitable barriers to communication can, in fact, actually make matters worse. If cultural differences are more aptly viewed as 'ethnic markers', treating these differences as objective 'facts' getting in the way of good health care may simply furnish professionals with an alibi for inadequacies and shortcomings which have quite different origins (see Van Dijk, 1998).

3.3. Sociological approaches

Transcultural mental health care is currently strongly influenced by anthropology, but medical sociology also contains concepts that have contributed to critical thinking about the care of refugees. Two important notions are 'the social construction of illness' and the importance of power relations in health care.

3.3.1. The social construction of illness

The notion of illness as a social construction was already implicit in the 'new transcultural psychiatry'. Kleinman (1988) criticized what he called the 'pathogenic / pathoplastic' model, in which biological factors *determine the form* of an illness, while cultural factors merely *influence its content*. This model, which De Jong (1996) wittily dubbed the 'striptease model' of illness, is implicit in the WHO's epidemiological studies and in many notions of 'cultural sensitivity'. As we saw above, illnesses (according to present-day transcultural psychiatrists) are inextricably rooted in a cultural context, so that it makes no sense to regard cultural factors as 'secondary'.

Within medical sociology, the notion of 'illness as a social construct' (cf. Wright & Treacher, 1982) has its roots not in interpretative anthropology, but in symbolic interactionism. The two approaches share many presuppositions in common, but tend to be academically separate. In positivist medicine and psychology, it is assumed that illnesses have an objective existence regardless of the way we think about them. Psychiatrists *discover* illnesses, just as botanists discover plant species. The notion of social construction, however, implies that illnesses are not so much discovered as *invented*. They come into being within a particular way of framing experience and cannot meaningfully be said to exist outside of that framework.

The concept of 'trauma' has been a favorite target of attention for social constructionists. In an oft-quoted passage, Allan Young (1995, p. 5) wrote:

> The disorder is not timeless, nor does it possess an intrinsic unity. Rather, it is glued together by the practices, technologies, and narratives with which it is diagnosed, studied, treated, and presented by the various interests, institutions, and moral arguments that mobilized these efforts and resources.

The sudden rise of the trauma concept in the 1980s in the context of a dispute about the compensation of Vietnam veterans makes it an ideal candidate for such an analysis. Those who believe 'trauma' exists independently of the way people think about it, regard it as simply a new name for a phenomenon that has long been recognized under labels such as 'railway spine' or 'shell shock'. If 'trauma' is a quasi-biological phenomenon whose essence lies outside culture, then it is logical to assume that the concept developed for dealing with U.S. service personnel will be equally useful for categorizing victims of organized violence all over the world – indeed, throughout history.

An example of the objections to this view is given by Jones et al. (2003). These authors argue, on the basis of an extensive analysis of patient records, that 'flashbacks' – a crucial ingredient of PTSD – were virtually unknown in previous wars. If we view 'trauma' as a social construct, there is no *a priori* reason to expect it to be the most relevant or the most fruitful concept to apply to a particular group of refugees. Of course, it *is* routinely applied to such groups and often functions as the basis for service delivery – but that is not to say that other concepts, specifically tailored to the groups in question, would not do the job better.

However, two caveats need to be applied to the social constructionist approach. Firstly, it must not be forgotten that saying an illness is 'invented' does not mean that it is *fictitious* – that those claiming to suffer from it are not 'really' ill. An illness concept is a way of framing experiences, and those experiences may be as harrowing and severely handicapping as any. To regard an illness as a 'social construction' is not to say that all those with the diagnosis are simply malingering.

Secondly, following on from this point, we should bear in mind that a diagnosis has important social and legal consequences as well as medical ones. Regarding 'trauma' (or 'anorexia', or 'hyperactivity') as a social construction may be misinterpreted as implying that it is not 'real' and that all such diagnoses are mistaken. This misunderstanding can have disastrous consequences for the people whose pension rights or asylum status are jeopardized by it (cf. Watters, 2001, p. 1710).

An analogy may be instructive here. In the hey-day of coal mining, a diagnosis of 'miner's nystagmus' was the royal road to compensation for incapacitated miners. By the 1930's, this disorder had become in Britain the most important item of compensation in the mining industry. Carl Figlio's (1982) social-constructionist account of this diagnosis shows much resemblance to the story of PTSD. For example, the link between the central symptom of nystagmus (oscillatory movements of the eyes) and incapacitation was actually quite weak. Nystagmus had above all a *symbolic* function: it was the emblem of a 'deserving case'. For all that, few people today would deny the right of those miners to their money. Likewise, a PTSD diagnosis is the royal road to compensation for victims of many different sorts of violence, including refugees, and until a better system can be devised it would be wrong and until a better system can be devised it would surely be unjust to block off this road[7].

Perhaps these considerations can provide a key to understanding the spectacular rise in popularity of the PTSD concept. In section 3.1, I referred to this popularity as a 'riddle': how could a concept which so inadequately describes the hardships refugees are

---

[7] In this connection we may note that the critical study by Jones et al. (2003) was financed by the US Army.

exposed to, and the problems these give rise to, have enjoyed such success? In my view, the answer has mainly to do with the *social consequences* of a diagnosis of PTSD.

Experience has shown that legal agencies, government departments and insurance companies tend to be unimpressed by problems formulated in terms of the approaches which we characterized in section 3.1 as 'soft'. Phenomenological, holistic accounts paying regard to social context, meaning and illness experience, however indispensable they may be for effective care delivery, do not get you very far in a court of law: a clever lawyer can demolish such an account in no time. Far more suited to this arena are the categorical, black-and-white descriptions which characterize the 'biomedical' approach, in which a fundamental distinction is assumed between normality and pathology.

A recent example illustrates this clearly. At the beginning of 2003 a Congolese asylum seeker, Jean-Claude Mputu-Bola, was refused asylum on humanitarian grounds by the British government. His request for political asylum had been turned down because his accounts of mistreatment and torture in Angola failed to convince government investigators, who also regarded the country as a safe place for him to return to. Subsequently, asylum on humanitarian grounds was requested on the grounds that he was severely depressed as a result of his sister's having been tortured to death after being found in possession of a letter from him. However, this request was turned down because, in the words of the Home Office, depression would be *'understandable in one so far away from his family who has seen grim sights'* (source: NCADC, 2003; my italics).

This example shows that the effects of concepts in a judicial setting are quite different from their application in a care setting. Many mental health workers strive to avoid 'pathologizing' or 'medicalizing' their client's problems and try to blur the distinction between normality and pathology. However, this 'normalizing' approach (Ingleby, 1980), which emphasizes that many supposed forms of pathology are 'understandable' in everyday terms, can be disastrous in a court of law. Managers of mental health services are another group with a traditional preference for the cut and dried, no-nonsense character of biomedical concepts. Indeed, the need to agree on a framework for setting treatment costs was one of the main considerations underlying the introduction of the DSM as a universal frame of reference for mental health services.

So we see that it is no accident that PTSD, a limited and by no means representative example of the problems refugees may have, acquired such a special status. Like the example of miner's nystagmus discussed earlier, it functions as an *emblem* for the effects of organized violence, as a key which can open certain doors. At the present time, the same phenomenon can be observed in two other areas:

- Large numbers of young women show various kinds of *eating disorders,* but the concept of 'anorexia nervosa'- which is strictly speaking only applicable to a tiny minority of all cases – has acquired the status of emblem for this group (see Schoemaker, 2002).
- Among boys, many kinds of *conduct disorders* cause considerable problems for themselves and others. However, these problems tend not to get taken very seriously unless the child is regarded as suffering from ADHD (attention deficit hyperactivity disorder). Again, very few children with conduct disorders actually conform to the diagnostic criteria for ADHD.

Characteristic of these four diagnoses – nystagmus, PTSD, anorexia and ADHD – is that they are liberally applied (respectively) to miners, refugees, young women and boys, mostly without a rigorous diagnostic procedure being followed. What I have tried to make clear in this section is that this should not be dismissed as mere exaggeration: such a label is an important way – sometimes, the only way – to get something done about the underlying problems.

3.3.2. The sick role: illness and power

The social consequences of 'having PTSD' are an illustration of the American sociologist Talcott Parsons' theory of the sick role. Ascription of sickness does not simply indicate what is going on inside your body: as we have just seen, it redefines your rights and your place in society. Critics of what they regard as excessive diagnosis accuse professionals of 'medicalizing' human difficulties or deviance, with the effect of stigmatizing people and consigning them to the role of passive victims who have lost control of their lives. According to this view, those concerned may often simply be reacting in a normal way to abnormal experiences or situations. Though the status of 'victim' may help in obtaining political asylum, it can create an extra handicap when it comes to social integration. Opponents of medicalization therefore insist on using the term 'survivor' for those who have experienced violence; they prefer to describe help as 'empowerment' rather than 'treatment' (see Chapter 9 by Choman Hardi).

This discussion is centered on issues of *power,* a concept which does not figure in purely biomedical models. Such models ignore, in particular, the power of the health professionals themselves: these workers are seen as performing a purely technical task, whose necessity is self-evident. Yet professions are not purely idealistic organizations without any interests of their own. They form, in Freidson's (1970) words, a 'labor market shelter', with an inherent interest in delineating, claiming and controlling a market. These activities are sometimes referred to as 'professional imperialism'. An enormous expansion of the demand for trauma therapy, for example, redistributes the *economic* power of the different caring professions and also shifts the balance of power between professionals and the public. The term 'trauma industry', coined in reaction to the spectacular rise of the concept after 1980, is not just a disparaging metaphor but points to important political and economic realities.

3.4. Managed care

An increasingly important factor influencing service provision in the last two decades has been changing approaches to care management. In Western countries, the phenomenon of 'managed care' has arisen in response to the enormously increased demand for health services of all kinds. Governments and insurance companies that financed these services urgently needed to find ways of controlling costs and increasing efficiency. To this end, management techniques and personnel were imported from other sectors and organizations, the assumption being that principles of good management were universal.

This increase in the power of managers caused much resentment among health care workers, who saw their professional autonomy being whittled away by functionaries who might have no medical or psychological knowledge whatsoever. Management principles typically dictate an increase in the size of organizations through reorganizations, fusions and closures. The large agglomerations which came into being in this way were criticized as being 'impersonal' and 'monolithic'. A second principle of managed care was the 'rationalization' of treatment procedures. Standardized procedures for diagnosis and treatment were introduced which made it easier to quantify and monitor 'input' and 'output', but diminished still further the autonomy of the individual health worker.

Rationalization also influenced the *type* of information collected on clients. Checklists of symptoms which could be easily coded in digital form acquired priority over complex, contextualised narratives, in which human intuition or professional experience played a part. Unfortunately, standardized protocols for diagnosis and treatment presuppose standard clients, and this approach pays little attention to individual differences. Nor does it recognize the importance of *group differences,* such as cultural variations in the way problems are experienced and expressed. No allowance is made for the additional work of getting to know and understand clients with different cultural backgrounds. In this sense, rationalization has thus hampered the provision of 'culturally sensitive care'.

Yet there is another side to modern management approaches, which has actually been very useful for those trying to improve service provision for minority groups. The emphasis on *quality* and *quality control* gives these approaches, in theory at least, an inherently critical character. 'Managed care' has toppled many idols from their pedestals: treatments which could not produce evidence of their own effectiveness, institutions which refused to look critically at their traditions and cultures, professionals who subjected patients to their own fads or out-of-date knowledge – in principle, all of these could be undermined by the simple means of cutting off the money supply. There are important shortcomings in the way 'quality control' is presently operationalized, in particular the equation of 'evidence-based' approaches with quantitative methods of evaluation. The applicability of quantitative methods, especially in cross-cultural research, is actually quite limited. However, the notion of 'quality control' itself is an important stimulus to change in service provision, and the notion of 'good practice' is probably here to stay.

Moreover, some modern philosophies of health care management place an emphasis on the contribution of users which is totally at odds with the traditional 'top-down' culture of health care institutions. To ensure quality, service providers must look at their activities from the users' viewpoint. Do the services make sense to users? Do they inspire confidence and get people involved in their own recovery? How accessible are they? Usually, feedback from users is confined to a "patients' platform", but this excludes those for whom the service provision is so poorly designed that they never even come into contact with it.

If services have to be adapted ('tailor-made') to suit the needs of users, then it is inevitable that users must be more closely consulted about how this should be done. Effective services must therefore be 'user-led' rather than 'service-led'. In this respect, some strands of management philosophy agree in their conclusion with the multicultural health care movement discussed in the last section and the 'self-help' movement discussed in the following one.

3.5. The role of users' movements

Advocates of a 'self-help' approach often base their approach on the critique of 'professional imperialism' described above and focus particularly on the issues of power involved in handing over problems to professionals. They are, in other words, deeply ambivalent about the professionalization of human problems and promote as much as possible the solution of problems by the group itself.

Most self-help groups are intended for sufferers from a particular condition and/or their relatives. This focus on a particular diagnostic category ties them in, whether they like it or not, with the health care system. Other groups, however, arise within minority communities or special groups whose needs are not felt to be met by existing services. Their activities are typically directed towards 'empowerment' and 'advocacy' (lobbying and campaigning for the interests of their members).

In recent years, these groups have found an unexpected ally in policy makers who argue that users should have a hand in designing their own services. Sometimes the innovations they develop are indeed taken up and incorporated into 'the system'. Among the most successful examples have been women's groups or immigrant groups providing alternative services for specific needs. However, many refugees (especially asylum seekers) are handicapped by their insecure and transitory existence when it comes to forming their own organizations. Partly because of this, we see that most NGO's working for refugees are not themselves staffed by refugees (though some make an effort to rectify this situation). In spite of these disadvantages, a number of self-help organizations for refugees do exist.

Although there are hardly any countries in which asylum seekers and refugees have much influence in the design of their own service provisions, a comparative study carried out for the European Commission (see Chapter 12) revealed some interesting international differences. Compared with the British care system, the Dutch system emerged as a highly regulated, tightly-knit and somewhat closed system, allowing little room for initiatives or influences from outside groups. This may account for the fact that user involvement is much more in evidence in the UK than in The Netherlands.

One way in which users can influence the design of services, apart from through users' groups, is through their contribution to research. However, most research studies, because of their methodology, give a very limited opportunity for refugees and asylum seekers to describe their needs and problems in their own terms. This is because they make use of standardized questionnaires or diagnostic procedures, instead of methods which have more the character of a dialogue and allow the person interviewed to express themselves in their own way. Only field work using qualitative methods is capable of bringing the users' own perspective into focus. Ahearn (2000) describes the methodological dilemmas of research in this area. Such methods are seldom used within the health care system, though Sander Kramer describes in Chapter 8 a series of studies which have specifically set out to explore users' perspectives.

REFERENCES

Ahearn, F. L. (ed.) (2000) *Psychosocial wellness of refugees: issues in qualitative and quantitative research.* New York and Oxford: Berghahn Books.

Angel, B., Hjern, A. & Ingleby, D. (2001) Effects of war and organized violence on children: A study of Bosnian refugees in Sweden. *American Journal of Orthopsychiatry 71,* 4-15.

Barth, F. (ed.) (1969) E*thnic Groups and Boundaries: the social organization of cultural difference.* London: George Allen & Unwin

CSP (2003) *Global Conflict Trends.* Severn, MD: Center for Systemic Peace. http://members.aol.com/CSPmgm/conflict.htm

De Jong, J. (1996) Psychodiagnostiek met behulp van DSM of ICD: classificeren of nuanceren? In De Jong, J. & Van den Berg, M. (eds.), *Transculturele psychiatrie en psychotherapie. Handboek voor hulpverlening en beleid.* Amsterdam/Lisse: Swets & Zeitlinger.

De Jong, K., Mulhern, M., Ford, N., van der Kam, S., Kleber, R. (2000) The trauma of war in Sierra Leone. *Lancet 355,* 2067-70.

De Jong, K. (2001) Uses and abuses of the concept of trauma: a response to Summerfield. In Loughry, M. & Ager, A. (eds,), *Refugee Experience - Psychosocial Training Module.* Oxford: Refugee Studies Centre, 129-132.

Figlio, C. (1982) How does illness mediate social relations? Workmen's compensation and medico-legal practices, 1890-1940. In Wright, P. & Treacher, A. (eds.), *The problem of medical knowledge. Examining the social construction of medicine.* Edinburgh: Edinburgh University Press.

Freidson, E. (1970) *Profession of medicine. A Study of the Sociology of Applied Knowledge.* Chicago: Chicago University Press.

Garmezy, N. (1985). Stress-resistant children: the search for protective factors. In Stevenson, J. E (ed.), *Recent Research in Developmental Psychopathology.* Oxford, UK: Pergamon Press, 213-233.

Geertz, C. (1973) *The interpretation of cultures.* New York: Basic Books.

Gleditsch, N. P., Wallensteen, P., Eriksson, M., Sollenberg. M. & Strand, H. (2002) Armed Conflict 1946–2001: A New Dataset. *Journal of Peace Research 39,* 615–637. http://www.prio.no/cwp/ArmedConflict/

Ingleby, D. (ed.) (1980) *Critical Psychiatry. The Politics of Mental Health.* New York: Pantheon. Second impression, London: Free Association Books, 2004.

Ingleby, D. (2001) Asylum policies: part of the solution or part of the problem? Keynote address to the VIth International Conference for Health and Human Rights. Cavtat, Croatia, 21-24 June 2001. http://www.ishhr.org/conference/day_2_index.php

International Study Team (2003) *Our common responsibility: The impact of a new war on Iraqi children.* Toronto: War Child Canada.

Jones, E., Vermaas, R. H., McCartney, H., Beech, C., Palmer, I., Hyams, K. & Wesseley, S. (2003) Flashbacks and post-traumatic stress disorder: the genesis of a 20th-century diagnosis. *British Journal of Psychiatry 182,* 158-163.

Keilson, H., & Sarphatie, R. (1979). *Sequentielle Traumatisierung bei Kindern.* Stuttgart: Enke Verlag.

Kessler, R. C., Sonnega, A., Bromet, E,. Hughes, M. & Nelson, C. B. (1995) Posttraumatic stress disorder in the National Comorbidity Survey. *Archives of General Psychiatry 52,* 1048-1060.

Kleber, R. J., Brom, D., & Defares, P. B. (1992). *Coping with trauma: Theory, prevention and treatment.* Amsterdam/Berwyn, Pennsylvania: Swets and Zeitlinger International.

Kleber, R. J., Figley, C. R. & Gersons, B. P. R. (eds.) (1995) *Beyond trauma: cultural and societal dynamics.* New York, Plenum Press.

Kleinman, A., Eisenberg, L., & Good, B. (1978) Culture, illness, and care. Clinical lessons from anthropologic and cross-cultural research. *Annals of Internal Medicine 88,* 251-8.

Kleinman, A. (1981) *Patients and healers in the context of culture: an exploration of the borderland between anthropology, medicine and psychiatry.* Berkeley, CA: University of California Press.

Kleinman, A. (1988) *Rethinking psychiatry: From cultural category to personal experience.* New York: The Free Press.

Kraepelin, E. (1904) Vergleichende psychiatrie. *Zentralblatt für Nervenheilkunde und Psychiatrie 15,* 433–437.

Lazarus, R. S. & Folkman, S. (1984). *Stress, appraisal and coping.* New York: Springer.

Littlewood, R. (1990). From categories to contexts: a decade of the 'new transcultural psychiatry'. *British Journal of Psychiatry 156,* 308-23.

Marsella, A. J., Friedman, M. J., Gerrity, E. T. & Scurfield, R. M. (eds.) (1996) *Ethnocultural aspects of post-traumatic stress disorder: issues, research, and clinical applications*. Washington, D.C.: American Psychological Association.

Marshall, M. G. (2002) Measuring the Societal Impact of War. Chapter 4 in Fen Osler Hampson and David M. Malone (eds.), *From Reaction to Conflict Prevention: Opportunities for the UN System*. Boulder, CO: Lynne Rienner.

Marshall, M. G. & Gurr, T. R. (2003) *A global survey of armed conflicts, self-determination movements, and democracy*. Maryland, MD: Integrated Network for Societal Conflict Research (INSCR), Center for International Development and Conflict Management (CIDCM).
http://www.cidcm.umd.edu/inscr/peace.htm

NCADC (2003) Newsletter 13 February 2003. Manchester: National Coalition of Anti-Deportation Campaigns.

Robben, A. C. G. M. & Suárez-Oroczo, M. M. (eds.) (2000) Cultures under siege: collective violence and trauma. Cambridge: Cambridge University Press.

Rutter, M. (1987). Psychological resilience and protective mechanisms. *American Journal of Orthopsychiatry*, 45, 486-495.

Schoemaker, C. (2002) *Anorexia bestaat niet: het beeld van anorexia nervosa in de media*. Amsterdam: Archipel.

Silove, D. (1999) The psychosocial effects of torture, mass human rights violations, and refugee traumas. *Journal of Nervous and Mental Disease, 187*, 200-207.

Silove, D., Steel, Z. & Watters, C. (2000) Policies of deterrence and the mental health of asylum seekers. *Journal of the American Medical Association*, 284, 604-611.

Summerfield, D. (1995) Addressing human response to war and atrocity: major challenges in research and practices and the limitations of Western psychiatric models. In Kleber, R. J., Figley, C. R. & Gersons, B. P. R. (eds.) *Beyond trauma: cultural and societal dynamics*. New York, Plenum Press.

Summerfield, D. (1999) A critique of seven assumptions behind psychological trauma programmes in war-affected areas. *Social Science and Medicine 48*, 1449-1462.

Summerfield, D. (2001) The invention of post-traumatic stress disorder and the social usefulness of a psychiatric category. *British Medical Journal 322*, 95-98.

Summerfield, D. (2002) Mental health of refugees and asylum-seekers. Commentary. *Advances in Psychiatric Treatment*, 8, 247-8.

Turner, S., Bowie, C., Dunn, G., Shapo, L. & Yule, W. (2003) Mental health of Kosovan Albanian refugees in the UK. *British Journal of Psychiatry*, 182, 444-448.

UNHCR (2004) *Asylum Levels and Trends in Industrialized Countries, January - November 2003*. Geneva: United Nations High Commissioner for Refugees. www.unhcr.ch

USCR (2004) *World Refugee Survey 2004*. Washington, DC: U.S. Committee for Refugees.
www.refugees.org/WRS2004.cfm.htm

Van Dijk, R. (1996). Gedwongen migratie: kern van het vluchtelingenbestaan. In De Jong, J. & Van den Berg, M. (eds.), *Transculturele psychiatrie en psychotherapie. Handboek voor hulpverlening en beleid*. Amsterdam/Lisse: Swets & Zeitlinger, 21-34.

Van Dijk, R. (1998) Culture as excuse. The failures of health care to migrants in the Netherlands. In Van der Geest, S. & Rienks, A. (eds.), *The art of medical anthropology. Readings* (243-251). Amsterdam: Spinhuis.

Van Willigen, L. H. M. & Hondius, A. J. K. (1992) *Vluchtelingen en gezondheid*. Amsterdam/Lisse: Swets & Zeitlinger.

Van Willigen, L. H. M. (ed.) (2000) *Health hazards of organized violence in children II – Coping and Protective Factors*. Utrecht: Pharos.

Van Willigen, L. H. M. (2003) *Gevluchte kinderen – preventie van ziekte en bevordering van gezondheid*. Ede: Stichting MOA Oost Nederland.

Watters, C. (2001) Emerging paradigms in the mental health care of refugees. *Social science and medicine, 52*, 1709-1718.

Wright, P. & Treacher, A. (eds.) (1982) *The problem of medical knowledge. Examining the social construction of medicine*. Edinburgh: Edinburgh University Press.

Yehuda, R. (2003) Changes in the concept of PTSD and trauma. *Psychiatric Times 10*, 1-5.

Young, A. (1995) *The harmony of illusions. Inventing post-traumatic stress disorder*. Princeton, NJ: Princeton University Press.

Young, A. (2002) PTSD, Traumatic Memory and the Lessons of History. Paper presented at the Conference on Trauma, Culture and the Brain, Los Angeles.

2. FROM TRAUMA TO SURVIVAL AND ADAPTATION:
Towards a framework for guiding mental health initiatives in post-conflict societies

Derrick Silove[1]

Controversy continues about the value of implementing Western-based mental health interventions in societies emerging from mass conflict and displacement (Summerfield, 1999; Silove et al., 2000). Issues surrounding posttraumatic stress disorder (PTSD) have tended to dominate the debate with concerns being raised that the impact of psychic trauma has been overestimated (Summerfield, 1999) and that a singular focus on traumatic stress may divert attention from other pressing issues, particularly the plight of the severely mentally ill (Silove et al., 2000). The contentious debate about trauma (Summerfield, 1997a; de Vries, 1998) risks confusing donors, UN agencies and non-government organizations (NGO's) in the field, and may have the unintended effect of weakening the capacity of mental health professionals to contribute meaningfully to the relief effort.

A useful starting point in searching for a synthesis amongst competing viewpoints may be to describe briefly the three broad conceptual frameworks that inform most thinking in the field, namely the trauma, severe mental illness and psychosocial models, respectively. In what follows, a brief evaluation of the strengths and limitations of each model will be offered. In order to consider which aspects of these models may contribute most usefully to the relief and reconstruction effort, it is necessary first to consider the overall mission of international humanitarian aid programs (Sirleaf, 1993). Drawing on personal experiences, especially in Africa and in East Timor, I will highlight what I consider to be two key priorities of relief activities, namely to promote the capacity for survival (Davis, 1996) and for adaptation (Silove, 1999), a focus that may provide the basis for reconciling some of the conflicting perspectives that continue to dog the mental health field.

[1] Derrick Silove, Psychiatry Research and Teaching Unit, University of New South Wales, Sydney, Australia.

1. EMERGENCY HUMANITARIAN RELIEF, RECONSTRUCTION AND DEVELOPMENT

Distinctions have been drawn between the principles underlying emergency relief initiatives and programs that focus on reconstruction and development (Cuny, 1983; Middleton, 1998; Sirleaf, 1993). In reality, in many contemporary settings of chronic or recurrent conflict such as in Africa, in Asia, and in the Middle East, elements of both emergency and development programs need to be pursued concurrently, even if there may be some tensions about which approach should be given priority (van Damme, 1998b). For clarity, a simplified account of the two phases of international aid will be provided with the aim of identifying how mental health initiatives may form an integral part of each activity.

The primary purpose of emergency humanitarian relief operations, especially in the crisis or early post-crisis phase, is relatively simple: to maximize survival and to minimize harm by providing protection for as many vulnerable persons as possible (van Damme, 1998a; Davis, 1996). While the aim may be clear, the process whereby such initiatives are designed and orchestrated is extremely complex, with major challenges facing UN and other agencies in implementing an effective, unified and coherent strategy (Stubbs & Soroya, 1996) in a context where a multitude of organizations are active and where there is rapid flux in the social, political and security situation. Donors, United Nations agencies, international and local non-government organizations, political factions, and a myriad of religious, ethnic, and regional influences all play their roles in shaping the process. Forging a common purpose, coordinating efforts, preventing duplication of programs and ensuring that coherent goals are achieved, all can present formidable challenges. At worst, external aid may be manipulated in ways that foster conflict rather than peace (Harrell-Bond, 1986). In addition, needs that may seem easy to assess often prove to be difficult to gauge accurately. For example, predicting the extent and urgency of nutritional needs in different sectors of a disaster-affected population may prove to be a difficult undertaking (Sen, 1990), with inaccuracies in biometrics measurements, misrepresentation of needs, corruption, and political interference all potentially undermining the process (van Damme, 1998a).

Yet in some acute crises, the imperative to secure the survival of the population can be overriding, at times justifying rapid and decisive action based on an imperfect assessment of the situation. During a short time period of a few weeks in September 1999, most of the population of East Timor was displaced and militia supported by the Indonesian military destroyed more than 70% of the built and agricultural infrastructure of the territory. Locating and then providing food, water, shelter, emergency medical treatment and protection for over 600,000 persons spread over a mountainous and inaccessible terrain proved to be a daunting logistic challenge. As a consequence, at least in the early phases of such emergencies, a 'top-down' utilitarian strategy may be legitimate (van Damme, 1998a), with experts, usually imported from outside the arena of conflict, acting decisively with whatever technological support is available, to provide protection to large numbers of persons at risk of immediate harm. When the threat to the whole population is so acute, it is usually not possible, nor desirable, to attempt to undertake detailed and systematic needs assessments before acting – experts usually can make rapid global assessments based on past experience and available knowledge of the history and context of the conflict. More important is making accurate logistic assessments about how best to provide aid to those at greatest risk.

In the hierarchy of needs, the imperative to achieve physical survival and minimize harm for the maximum number of persons must take priority. It is self-evident that mass conflict leads to death, injury and physical disability (Toole & Waldman, 1988), but it is also true that many persons die in the post-conflict phase – often the cause is obvious (injury, infectious diseases, malnutrition) (Toole & Waldman, 1990). However, in many instances the reasons are more obscure (Eitinger & Strom, 1973), raising the possibility that an ill-defined subgroup die or are injured, not directly as a consequence of warfare, but because of one or more interrelated behavioral disturbances such as risk taking, misadventure, impaired judgment, homicide and/or suicide.

The 'culture' of urgency that is generated in acute emergencies can produce makeshift and clumsy solutions such as the confinement of large numbers of persons in refugee camps (van Damme, 1995) and the forced separation of men from women and children, strategies which, in the short term, may assist the goal of achieving maximal protection, but that, in the medium to long-term, may have adverse psychosocial consequences by disrupting traditional social groupings and perpetuating an ethos of helplessness and passivity in the population (Silove, 1995). Although intended as a temporary protection strategy, such a dependency model inadvertently can become chronic where communities remain confined for decades in refugee camps and detention centers.

How can professionals mount a credible case that mental health activities should be given some priority in a context where life and death issues are paramount? I will attempt to develop the argument throughout this text that the opportunity for mental health professionals to make a meaningful contribution, especially in the immediate post-emergency phase, lies in their ability to enhance the overall goal of enhancing the survival capacity of vulnerable sectors of the population, especially if the subsidiary aim is to assist in creating a protection regime that fosters the human rights and dignity of all affected persons.

Development aid focuses more on a medium and long-term perspective. Sen (1989; 1999a) has pointed out that development cannot be measured in strict economic terms, but that it has to encompass the broader task of expanding human capabilities and promoting freedom in a context of social responsibility. Hence, there is increasing recognition that genuine and sustainable development of societies disrupted by war and conflict can only occur if the impetus and leadership for such initiatives comes from within the community itself. Capacity building and sustainability of programs (Reinke et al., 1997) thus have become the cornerstones of development aid since these principles encourage a focus on skills enhancement, community participation, the promotion of leadership, and the creation of an ethos of communal self-reliance and self-determination.

Although these principles are easy to comprehend, the way they are interpreted and implemented is not always free of ambiguity. In a society that is grossly disrupted by mass conflict and where resources are limited, it is not always clear who should determine which capacity should be developed and to what end. The intermingling of the emergency and reconstruction phases, especially in situations of low-grade civil war, invariably creates tensions between the imperative of meeting survival need and the priority of developing durable structures and programs that will promote participation and autonomy (van Damme, 1998b).

There is a risk in the post-emergency phase that the sense of urgency will encourage mental health experts in the field to attempt to achieve rapid results in domains that are not amenable to such outcomes. Some capacities in health service provision can be developed rapidly, but others, particularly in mental health, may require a graduated approach in order to achieve a durable and self-sustaining skills base over time. In particular, questions remain about claims that the local population can be given brief training and then rapidly mobilized across a chaotic environment, not only to work as mental health workers but also to train others in the acquired skills (the train-the-trainer model). The risks to trainees and recipient communities of applying such an oversimplified model of intervention will be referred to below. Furthermore, brief community-wide interventions aimed at preventing the long-term impact of trauma, often referred to as 'debriefing' (Raphael & Wilson, 2000), remain controversial, even in Western settings (see below).

 In summary, in spite of the shortcomings of past efforts (Stubbs & Soroya, 1996), international intervention in humanitarian crises cannot always be avoided, especially where large numbers of a population may be at risk of death, injury and disability as a consequence of mass violence. Nevertheless, the social risks of such interventions are substantial – in particular, if poorly managed, programs can perpetuate dependency and alienation and set in place structures, such as refugee camps, that can become semi-permanent locations of confinement of large populations (Waldron, 1987).

As indicated, the precise role of mental health initiatives within this broader framework of humanitarian aid and development still need to be settled. Across many societies, the status of psychiatry and mental health remain controversial, with a strong tendency – observed across many cultures- to ridicule, dismiss or marginalize those afflicted by psychological disturbances. Such a tendency may be magnified in post-conflict settings where the urgency of survival needs and the scarcity of resources may encourage key health and administrative personnel to assign low priority to mental health. It is vital therefore to consider how mental health programs can be harmonized with the overlapping missions of emergency aid and development. The extent to which strategies aim at supporting the central purpose of each phase – survival capacity in the emergency phase and adaptive capacity in the development phase- may prove to be the yardsticks against which mental health initiatives are judged. It is against this background that prevailing models of mental health will be considered.

2. MODELS OF MENTAL HEALTH

2.1. The Trauma Model

As indicated, controversy about the impact of psychic trauma on populations exposed to mass violence and displacement has tended to dominate debate in the field, with two theoretical poles emerging (Silove et al., 2000) – at one extreme, protagonists of the conventional traumatology perspective have tended to highlight the pervasiveness of trauma and its psychological consequences in such settings (Agger et al., 1995), whereas detractors of the trauma model have cast doubt on whether diagnostic constructs such as PTSD have any meaning or salience in non-Western societies (Summerfield, 1999). The ensuing debate is important not only for theoretical reasons, but also because it may have important practical implications in shaping the priorities of those leaders entrusted with planning and implementing health and social programs in post-conflict societies.

The arguments underlying the critique of PTSD have been comprehensively explored by Summerfield and colleagues in several publications (Summerfield, 1997a; Summerfield, 1999) and will not be repeated in detail herein. In essence, objections have been raised about the tendency to describe entire populations as traumatized simply because they have lived through states of warfare and conflict; about the medicalization of normative expressions of suffering by imposing western-derived diagnostic entities such as PTSD on survivors; about the assumption that psychological reactions are as salient as the immediate practical survival and adaptive needs facing post-conflict societies; and about the risks of importing western derived counseling techniques into cultures and contexts where such interventions are alien and potentially undermining of communal strategies for social recovery (Silove, 2000b) .

No attempt will be made herein to provide a comprehensive rebuttal of this critique, not least because many of the concerns have a degree of legitimacy – in particular, the objection to the notion that large sectors of war-affected and displaced populations are traumatized and hence need intensive psychological assistance (Silove, 1999). At the same time, it is important not to overlook the advances that have been made in the study of traumatic stress in refugee and post-conflict populations (Mollica, 2000), knowledge that has provided an important corrective to the mass denial of psychological suffering that often accompanies humanitarian disasters (Raphael and Wilson, 2000). The capacity to record meaningful subcategories of trauma across cultures (Mollica, 2000), the development of instruments to measure both Western-derived and culture-specific responses to trauma (Mollica et al., 1992), and the demonstration that particular forms of abuse such as torture increase risk of detrimental psychological outcomes (Basoglu et al., 1994, Steel et al., 1999), together provide an important scientific foundation for a field that for too long has drawn much of its support from poorly founded rhetoric.

A major advance in research has been the application of rigorous epidemiological techniques to the study of the population-wide impact of gross human rights violations, war and displacement (Mollica et al., 1993; Mollica et al., 1999; Shrestha et al., 1998). By avoiding the biases of clinical or other convenient samples, these studies have been able to identify more accurately both the prevalence of common psychological reactions and the risk factors associated with these outcomes. Yet the results of these studies raise important questions that need to be addressed in future research, particularly in relation to the matching of needs to available expertise and resources. Most research studies have found that that the majority of war-affected populations survive without any long-term psychological disability (Silove, 1999). Nevertheless, recent studies indicate that PTSD affects a sizeable minority of persons with the average prevalence rate across studies being approximately 14% (Z. Steel, *personal communication*).

If such figures are accepted at face value, then the health implications are extensive – the implied need far exceed the potential for resource-poor communities to respond meaningfully to the problem, even with support from the outside world. Taken together, therefore, the findings of epidemiological studies on PTSD are at risk of provoking unintended reactions from the leaders of relief efforts whose task it is to make difficult decisions about allocating scarce resources – either the high rates of PTSD will be interpreted as reflecting normative reactions not warranting attention or, at the other extreme, legitimate objections will be raised about the wisdom of focusing on a problem of such magnitude that it defies any short-term solution.

2.1.1. A Pragmatic Perspective on Trauma

It is timely therefore to re-evaluate the implications of trauma research undertaken in post-conflict and refugee populations, not to reject the value of such epidemiological investigations, but rather to apply a more stringent and discriminatory approach to interpreting the findings, particularly in relation to matching the urgency of needs with available resources. In such a re-evaluation, several issues need to be considered. The prevalence of acute traumatic stress symptoms is high in any group recently exposed to life threatening trauma (Modvig et al., 2000). It should be noted that rates of PTSD vary substantially according to the criteria used and different methods for identifying the disorder produce significantly different prevalence rates (Fleming et al., 1999; Peters et al., 1999). Although problematic for epidemiologists, this observation does not necessarily present a particular challenge to the status of PTSD – the measurement of other psychiatric disorders is beset with similar problems. In addition, in most, early symptoms of PTSD will resolve spontaneously (Kessler et al., 1995), particularly if the environment is supportive. In particular, it is clear that the quality of the recovery environment contributes substantially to the outcome of early PTSD reactions (Steel et al., 1999) so that attention to issues of security and safety are paramount. Even in those whom PTSD persists, it is characteristic for symptoms to fluctuate over time. Hence, epidemiological studies focusing on a single measure of PTSD measured at one point in time, especially if undertaken in the immediate aftermath of a humanitarian disaster, are unlikely to provide accurate information about the urgency of treatment needed. Although groups at high risk to chronicity have been identified 'survivors of concentration camps, torture and sexual abuse' (Malt et al., 1996), and there are some characteristics that are associated with a good prognosis 'such as continuing engagement in political or religious activities' (Allden et al., 1996), the overall variability in the course of PTSD is so substantial that predicting the outcome in any individual case remains problematic, especially in the early phase after trauma exposure(Green, 1996).

The question of disability associated with PTSD thus becomes pivotal, since several authorities have noted that a substantial portion of persons with PTSD still may function effectively in spite of the presence of symptoms (Mollica et al., 1993; Summerfield, 1999). In contrast, studies are emerging to show that some persons with PTSD face long-term disability of a severe type (Kessler, 2000). A step forward in knowledge is the discovery that co-morbidity – the presence of PTSD and depression– is associated with much higher levels of disability in a refugee population (Mollica et al., 1998), a finding that has been replicated recently by our own team (Momartin, *personal communication*) and extended to show that such co-morbidity-related disability may persist for years after exposure to war trauma.

Help-seeking patterns also need to be considered in interpreting the practical implications of recent epidemiological studies on trauma. There is consistent evidence from the general epidemiological literature that even in western countries where services are readily accessible, only a portion of persons with psychiatric disorders seek treatment (Meltzer et al., 1995). In addition, it is well known that relatively few persons with PTSD seek professional help (Kessler, 2000) and some persons can show adverse reactions to treatment (Pitman et al., 1991). Treatment seeking depends on a complex interaction of symptom type and severity, coping and other factors associated with adaptation (Priebe and Esmaili, 1997). With the exception of a few treatments (medications, behavioral methods), doubts still persist about which of the extensive array of interventions offered for PTSD are effective and which are most readily adapted to different cultures and contexts (Silove, 1999).

In summary, progress towards a pragmatic epidemiology of traumatic stress reactions in post-conflict environments will be enhanced if the focus on measuring trauma reactions is matched with questions of urgency of need and feasibility of interventions. In that way, traumatologists will obviate the risk of emphasizing the ubiquity of traumatic stress at the expense of defining the core subgroup with severe trauma-related mental disabilities that require priority attention.

2.2. Severe Mental Illness

The plight of the severely mentally ill in post-conflict settings has attracted remarkably little attention (Silove et al., 2000). One of the reasons for this oversight may be the overweening preoccupation with trauma and PTSD referred to above. Another may be the concern, alluded to briefly earlier, that western models of mental illness may not be appropriate when applied unmodified to other cultures and contexts. In that respect, the transcultural mental health field appears to be divided into two opposing conceptual frameworks. The universalistic or "etic" position, ascribed to western psychiatry, assumes that core patterns of psychiatric illness can be identified, with minor variations, across cultures and contexts. In contradistinction, transculturalists steeped in the ethnographic or "emic" tradition tend to regard culture as playing a pivotal role both in the genesis and shaping of mental distress and in its expression (Minas and Silove, 2001).

Classification systems such as the Diagnostic and Statistical Manual, edition IV, have intensified the debate about cultural relevance and meaning. Such nosologies, although giving some recognition to cultural variations, tend to be largely universalistic in their formulations. At the same time, the emic position, if adopted in its most extreme form, has serious practical implications – if that formulation is correct, then it follows that western psychiatry has little to offer other cultures and may in fact do damage if imported uncritically into societies with diverse traditions of diagnosis and healing.

There are several issues that may temper the polar extremes of both the emic and etic perspectives respectively. There can be no doubt that there is substantial cultural variation in the understanding and expression of mental distress and in the explanatory models invoked to make sense of unusual behaviors across cultures (Kleinman, 1988; Kirmayer, 1989) – ignoring such context-based interpretations is likely to cause serious transcultural errors. Western treatments may be prescribed as a band-aid that obscures the social underpinnings of the underlying problem. For example, in a refugee camp in Africa, young women who collapse suddenly and remain unresponsive for some time often are diagnosed as hysterical and are routinely given injections of a tranquilizer, with recovery usually occurring within 12 hours. This medicalization of the problem does little to address the common underlying conflict – the woman's desperation at being forced into an arranged marriage with an older man.

At the same time, the tendency to regard traditional cultures as monolithic and unchanging although possibly still relevant to some small and isolated communities- can be overdrawn. Sen (1999b) has argued that the western perspective may underestimate the extent of heterodoxy in values and belief systems of Asian societies, a point he emphasizes by describing periods of cultural, religious and political pluralism in the history of India. In the present epoch, cultural change and interchange appears to be an irreversible reality whether or not mental health professionals play a role in that process. This change may be promoted excessively and exploited under the guise of globalization, a self-fulfilling prophecy that can inflict irreparable damage on local traditions and cultures. Nevertheless, how cultures can be protected from external influences, especially by mental health professionals, is far from clear – the argument for imposed isolation and neglect by outsiders seems to have no greater moral force than a considered and measured approach to intercultural engagement, as long as emphasis is given to establishing an ethos of mutual respect and partnership, and a willingness by both sides to learn from each other.

It also is important to acknowledge that even in the West, psychiatric classification is still largely based on a nominalist foundation – with the exception of the clearly defined organic disorders, almost all presently used diagnostic categories are, at best, provisional. No sufficient or even necessary causal factors have been identified, and there are no independent measures of validity for individual diagnostic categories. This contrasts with most illness categories in general medicine where the ability to isolate a specific organism, undertake a blood test, or examine a specimen of tissue, supports the presence of an underlying disease process. Hence, at present, the classification of mental disorders is based on a dialectical process in which diagnostic tradition, evolving theory, clinical consensus, and scientific research are combined (or compete) with political, social and utilitarian factors in determining whether particular categories are retained, added or deleted from existing nosologies – a decision usually made ultimately by an expert committee (Zarin & Earls, 1993). The mistake therefore is to reify the present system, a problem typified by the debate as to whether PTSD exists or not – in essence both sides of the debate are in error, since there is no critical test at present, either theoretical or concrete, to settle the question.

Importantly, there is a growing view in western psychiatry that the mental health system in general should focus less on the specifics of diagnosis and more on the social context and consequences of illness, particularly on issues of disability and incapacity (Hargreaves et al., 1984). This prescription from the general psychiatric literature may be of help in guiding transcultural practitioners through a middle path between the extreme emic and etic divide. In essence, a combination of indicators – ecological, social, familial, behavioral, subjective and cultural needs to be combined in making a contextually based assessment of any problem. In some instances, the local cultural judgment may be in error. An example is the case of a young woman in a refugee camp who was assumed to be mad because she screamed uncontrollably whenever she was in the vicinity of young men – in reality, this was a deliberate ploy to safeguard herself against the ever-present threat of rape which was rampant in the camp. In this context, being labeled mad conferred greater protection than being considered sane. In other instances, there may be a clear consensus across the cultural divide about the presence of mental illness and its threatening consequences – a brief case vignette illustrates this point.

Two western-trained mental health professionals working as consultants to the UN visited a refugee camp with 2,000 inhabitants on the Burundi border. There were no psychiatric services in the camp, but the officials in charge stated that they could identify approximately 70 persons in urgent need of psychiatric care. The mental health professionals were escorted to see one such person – a woman in her 30's living in squalor on the edge of the camp. She was described as acting bizarrely, screaming at non-existent figures and wandering around the camp in a disorganized fashion. As a consequence, she had become a social outcast, the target of derision and violence, including repeated sexual abuse by gangs of young men. She had lost two infants as a consequence of infection and malnutrition – the mother would not allow officials to assist her in their care. Further sexual abuse had produced another young infant whom the mother would not allow anyone to touch. When interviewed with an interpreter, it was clear, in spite of the language barrier, that the woman held persecutory beliefs (beyond the reality of her daily abuse by others) and was incoherent in her thinking. She laughed and giggled for no reason, appeared to be responding to auditory hallucinations, and was clearly disorganized in her handling of the infant. Physically, she was disheveled, emaciated and displayed scars and injuries from the abuse she had suffered. Suggestions that she might move to a special compound for at-risk persons met with physical resistance motivated, it seemed, by the woman's misunderstanding of the intentions of her helpers.

Whereas the mental health practitioner working in a transcultural setting may reserve judgment about the specific, context-based root causes of the mental disturbance, the general pattern of psychosis, recognized both by the local community and by the experts, as in the case described above, still may allow a broad case identification to be made and appropriate treatment to be instituted – especially where, as was the situation in the refugee camp, there were no traditional healers available. Such cultural and context-based failures in the capacity to care for specific sectors of the population are common in highly disrupted communities. Even when available, traditional healers can vary in the effectiveness of their ministrations – as in western medicine, there are charlatans interspersed among the true shamans. Cases I have reviewed in Africa and Cambodia of persons with psychosis revealed that some had been extensively burnt by traditional healers, others had been made extremely ill by herbs inducing vomiting and diarrhea, and one case had nearly asphyxiated from multiple seizures induced by a natural medicine.

In addition, stigma and marginalization of the severely mentally ill is common across many cultures – in parts of Africa, persons with epilepsy are regarded as being possessed and may be shunned to the point where they may not be assisted if overtaken by seizure, even if they fall into the fire. In times of civil war and mass displacement, those with established mental illnesses are made even more vulnerable to neglect, abandonment, abuse and exploitation (Silove et al., 2000). Institutions, including psychiatric facilities, often are destroyed or abandoned; leaving previously cared for patients without protection, medication or social support. Persons with overt psychosis may be found living in states of gross dereliction, often-falling prey to malnutrition, stigma, and ostracism. The mentally ill are at risk therefore to life threatening physical illness, death from misadventure or violence, and suicide. Children born of psychotic mothers, often as a consequence of rape, may be at high risk of death from malnutrition and disease resulting from maternal neglect. It is not unusual for mentally ill persons to be chained to trees or posts simply to prevent them from assaulting family members, from wandering, or from being attacked by neighbors or strangers. Having to contain a chronically mentally ill person may be the critical element that prevents a family unit from achieving some degree of self-sufficiency under already precarious conditions. Bizarre and disruptive social behavior by a few psychotic persons, when occurring repeatedly in a confined situation such as a refugee camp, can have an erosive impact on the already fragile social fabric of displaced communities.

Social networks and indigenous healing practices that may assist in the care of the mentally ill often are disrupted by war and displacement. Emergency health services provided by relief organizations rarely include psychiatrists so that personnel often are at a loss to know how to deal with persons with severe mental illnesses, and sufferers may be condemned to prolonged periods of time without access to appropriate treatment. Psychiatric medication is rarely available and even if some drugs are present, few personnel know how to prescribe them correctly. As a consequence, there can be an indiscriminate and overuse of minor tranquilizers which are potentially addictive and do little to relieve severe disorders such as psychosis and depression.

There is mounting evidence that efficient, low-technology, community-based mental health services can be established as part of the overall health program mounted in post-conflict societies (Silove et al., 2000). In all three sites with which I am familiar – the refugee camps of the Great Lakes region of Africa, a project run by the Harvard Program of Refugee Trauma in Cambodia, and the Program for Psychosocial Recovery and Development in East Timor (PRADET), a project of the University of New South Wales, substantial numbers of persons have attended the available services voluntarily, with some patients and their families traveling long distances to seek help. Many patients may have received traditional treatments suggesting a high level of pragmatism and hetero-doxy in the way people approach health care – ultimately, the most important concern is whether treatments work.

Impressive outcomes are often observed, especially as most persons are naïve to treatments, unlike the situation in the West where patients often pass through several hands. Persons confined to huts, tied to trees or left to wander at large may respond rapidly to standard treatments for psychosis or severe mood disturbances, thereby creating conditions, which allow the family and the wider network to re-engage the person in the process of care and rehabilitation. The economic impact on the family can be critical as illustrated by a case I reviewed in Cambodia. A young man, previously the most productive worker in the family's rice field, developed an acute psychosis and was chained to a tree for his own protection and that of his family. After receiving treatment from the newly established Harvard program, the man made substantial progress, and when visited by a review team, was found to be working industriously and seemingly free from symptoms in the rice field with his family.

Nevertheless, establishing such mental health programs in complex environments is not without its risks. For reasons of cost, the older psychiatric medications tend to be used even though they a have higher risk of adverse effects, some of which can be dangerous, especially in a setting where the patient's progress is difficult to monitor. Western-trained mental health staff inadvertently can undermine the work of traditional healers and it may prove difficult to foster an ethos of cooperation with this sector. Pressures may exist to develop structures, particularly inpatient facilities that replicate the worst legacies of western psychiatry – the isolation and institutionalization of the mentally ill. Once established, such institutions risk irreparably damaging the family's sense of responsibility to care for its members, a tradition that is ubiquitous in non-western societies. A warehousing mentality – the exclusion and confinement of the mentally ill – may supervene, inpatient institutions may drain the limited funds available for mental health, and a lack of resources and expertise increase the risk that such locations will become sites of neglect and abuse. Hence, it behooves mental health professionals to advocate strongly in favor of a decentralized, community-based approach for the development of mental health care in a context that actively involves the family and that ensures that the mentally ill are re-integrated into existing community life.

2.3. The Psychosocial Model

In recent times, increasing attention has focused on implementing what are broadly referred to as psychosocial programs of assistance for societies recovering from mass conflict. Such programs are supported by several principles: there is a diversity of needs in a society recovering from mass violence so that attention to the problems of the whole population provides maximal coverage; the psychosocial model is consistent with the aims of both emergency and development relief efforts in that it focuses on capacity building and community development; in their design, programs draw on the principles of public health by giving emphasis to health promotion, prevention and strategies of communal self-help; the focus is on forging partnerships, developing local leadership and fostering indigenous initiatives in repairing the social structure; much of the work is undertaken at the grassroots level, hence avoiding the need for expensive facilities or materials; reliance on external expertise and imported technology is minimized by involvement of local communities and personnel; programs can be designed to enhance cultural sensitivity and local traditions; and initiatives can be cost-saving in that they focus on whole population needs rather than on providing intensive aid to individuals.

Although these arguments are compelling, and are supported by policy initiatives of major international agencies, serious questions remain about the foundations on which the psychosocial model rests and about the practicalities of implementing wide-ranging programs. Although it is true that there is a diversity of psychosocial needs in post-conflict societies, it is equally true that not all needs are equally pressing. Comprehensive "need analyses", often undertaken as a preliminary to implementing psychosocial programs, are at risk of revealing too many needs and of demoralizing societies on which these analyses are undertaken. As a Sudanese headman living in a refugee camp remarked: 'They certainly must know what our needs are – they have come around with their questionnaires many times. We are still waiting for help!' Doubts remain as to whether broad-based psychosocial programs have any impact on those who are most disabled by traumatic stress and severe mental illness. Further, the scope and limits of programs are not always clear and issues remain about who is best equipped to undertake such initiatives. Most importantly, insufficient attention has been given to measuring and publishing project outcomes in a form that is easily accessible to an international audience.

The notion of rapid training and mobilization of indigenous community workers, a cornerstone of many programs, is particularly fraught in relation to mental health work, even of a preventive type. The necessary skills tend to be accrued incrementally over time, not only be direct didactic approaches, but also by supervision, mentoring and in-service training. The implementation of programs in complex and unstable environments is beset with risks and difficulties – worker burn out, cultural complexities, ethical and professional issues, and uncertainties about the effectiveness of strategies all suggest that care need to be taken in implementing and evaluating such programs. These issues can only be dealt with by a comprehensive approach to training with an effective system of support and supervision that is sustained over a reasonable period of time.

A further challenges to the psychosocial model is that programs often range over a wide territory, crossing boundaries between cultural, psychological, social, economic and human rights issues. Questions therefore arise as to the limits of psychological expertise needed in some programs. Raising awareness about mental health issues, establishing mental health associations and advocating for community participation in the development of mental health services are some of the community development activities that have concrete aims and outcomes. Conversely, strategies aimed at social reconstruction, those with experience in community development, legal or other skills may best implement reconciliation and justice.

Perhaps the greatest concern is the dearth of systematic evidence supporting the effectiveness of past programs. Such evidence needs to extend beyond expressions of satisfaction and gratitude by participating communities. However difficult, it is imperative that a body of data is generated to show with some objectivity that the community-wide aims of psychosocial programs are achieved and that the positive changes are sustained over time.

While the principles underlying the psychosocial model of intervention may be consistent with those driving the overall relief effort, much further attention needs to be given to questions of feasibility, practicality and outcomes. As will be argued below, with the restoration of safety, stability and material supplies, most individuals and their social structures are capable of making their own adaptations to the post-conflict situation without excessive external involvement. Programs that are clearly 'social' in their functions, in that they restore the fundamentals of communal life, may have greater legitimacy than those that attempt to have a direct psychological impact on a mass level, especially because many of those targeted will adapt naturally over time. At the same time, uncertainty persists as to the effectiveness of psychosocial programs in dealing with the minority who are severely disabled by posttraumatic stress disorders or severe mental illness.

3. A PROPOSED SURVIVAL AND ADAPTATIONAL FRAMEWORK

Based on the above considerations, a conceptual framework, adapted from previous work (Silove, 1999, Silove, 2000a) is offered to assist in guiding the focus of mental health initiatives in post-conflict societies. The framework is deliberately general in order to allow sufficient flexibility in the design and implementation of programs so that they match as closely as possible the specific context, culture and needs of individual societies recovering from mass conflict. The proposed "survival and adaptational model" aims to encompass elements of all three existing models in a way that promotes synergistic interactions amongst them. Importantly, the model attempts to bring coherence to the eclectic array of interventions that at present compete for priority in these settings.

Figures 1 and 2 outline the conceptual model proposed. It is based on the notion that, as the most evolved species on earth, human beings are adept at striving for survival and adapting to changing environments. The strategies they mount, either individually or collectively, are grounded in universal systems of behavior and social organization, although the form in which these activities are expressed is greatly influenced by culture and context. Hence, it is assumed that the core survival and adaptive systems that will be described have reciprocal representations in psychobiological substrates as well as in the social and cultural structures that humans create at the collective level.

Using the language of survival and adaptation assists in bringing the mental health enterprise closer to the objectives of the broader mission of emergency relief and social reconstruction following disasters. The model thus has important social and economic underpinnings: the repair and reconstruction of the physical and social environment is seen as crucial to, and in most instances sufficient to provide the basis for individuals and their communities to mobilize their own capacities for recovery and development. As a Timorese fisherman whose boats had been destroyed during the militia rampage in East Timor said to a visiting aid agency: 'Don't try to do the fishing for us. All we need are boats and nets and we will do our own fishing'.

The five survival and adaptive systems proposed in Figure 1 are hypothetical constructs that are considered to subsume the functions of 'safety', 'attachment', 'identity and role', 'justice', and 'existential meaning' (Silove, 1999). Although for simplicity, the systems identified are described separately, it is assumed that they have evolved in an orchestrated manner to ensure that, under normal circumstances, the interaction of the individual and his/her community occurs in a synergistic and mutually supportive way. In addition, the systems and the stresses that challenge them are not static but evolve over time. Thus threats may occur concurrently or sequentially, and their nature, meaning and impact may vary over time depending on the capacity of the individual and the group to adapt at key points in the process. Some challenges pose threats primarily to the survival capacity of the individual and the collective and others endanger long-term adaptation. Such distinctions are not absolute, however, with many challenges having impacts on both survival and adaptive capacities by exerting their influence across several of the identified systems.

3.1. The Security-Safety System

The core characteristic of man-made humanitarian crises is that they threaten the safety and security of the population (Figure 1). This reality, particularly in the emergency phase, is critical to guiding mental health priorities. Protection in these settings is fundamentally a social, political, and logistic activity, although the way it is implemented requires some understanding of mass psychology. Several subgroups in particular danger need mental health attention: those with severe mental illnesses exacerbated or provoked by the crisis; those with severe and disabling trauma reactions; those with physical injuries who have catastrophic psychological responses; those with brain injury or other nervous system disorders; and those with acute, culture-specific psychological reactions to stress.

The primary reason that aid workers and local leaders will seek assistance from mental health professionals, however, will be because of socially disruptive or disturbed behavior. This heterogeneous grouping will be referred to as the high-risk group. Although the group has certain features in common with those defined as the severely mentally ill in civil societies (Hargreaves et al., 1984), it is more inclusive and has special characteristics relevant to post-conflict settings. The most obvious subgroup includes those manifesting dangerous functioning – the suicidal, the homicidal, and those whose behaviors may place others at risk. The second subgroup comprises those who are gravely under-functioning, namely persons who, in spite of adequate opportunities, are not eating or drinking adequately, not attending to the most basic daily needs, or who are so irritable, distracted or immobilized as to place an unacceptable strain on the remainder of the family or group.

Figure 1. A survival and adaptation model

System	Challenge	Adaptive Response	Extreme Response	Social interventions	Psychological interventions	Psychiatric interventions
Security/ safety	Real threat (whole group)	Anxiety, security seeking	Terror, panic	Protection, curtailing hostilities	Crisis intervention for extreme reactions	
	Survival risk group (with mental disorders)	Good family and community care and protection	Dangerous or bizarre functioning, under-functioning. Extreme/ persistent distress	Special protection Support and education for family and network	Comprehensive assessment, crisis intervention, community follow-up, collaboration with traditional healers	Treat any underlying disorder (psychosis, severe depression, organic disturbances, etc)
	Persisting / excessive fear	Social and family support	Severe PTSD and related reactions	Maximize security and opportunities to regain control	Trauma counsel-ing: group or individual for selected few who are disabled	Adjunct psychiatric treatment for severe cases
Attach-ment	Ruptured bonds, mul-tiple losses & separations	Arousal, separation anxiety, grief	Prolonged or pathological grief, depression	Tracing and re-uniting families, Restoring social networks, rituals	Grief counseling for extreme reactions	Adjunctive treatment in minority with persisting /severe dysfunction
Justice	Human rights violations and abuses	Anger, frust-ration, caution in trusting; commitment to justice	Extreme anger	Truth, reconciliation, indictment, punishment, forgiveness	Group anger management in minority with persisting /severe dysfunction	Treat complications e.g. paranoia, depression in minority
Role/ identity	Disrupted institutions and structures	Role uncer-tainty / new roles and opportunities	Isolation, passivity, deviancy	Training, work, skills development	Elements of counseling/family therapy in severely affected	Adjunctive – for complications such as depression
Existen-tial meaning	Undermined values, culture and belief systems	Existential doubts. Adoption of new/hybrid identities	Alienation, Loss of faith	Religion, Political expression, cultural reconstruction	Elements of humanistic and existential therapy in counseling of severely disabled	Treat clinically severe depression

A sufficiently broad definition of survival should include the notion of survival with dignity so that those manifesting socially embarrassing and/or publicly bizarre behavior need to be attended to, for example, persons wandering around undressed in a crowded refugee camp, individuals drawing abuse or ridicule by virtue of their strange behavior, and persons who put themselves at health risk by uncharacteristic risk taking behavior such as promiscuity or heavy alcohol and drug use. The fourth and less clearly defined group are those whose social behavior, although not posing a direct threat to survival, clearly reflects an extreme level of suffering and distress that are not abating in spite of social measures to allay fear and insecurity – the humanitarian mission of aid programs clearly dictates that such persons should be given assistance. Members of this group, may be more difficult to identify – in a chaotic setting, the severely depressed who become withdrawn and suffer in silence may not attract attention.

Clearly, the urgency of need for this high-risk group (Figure 2) is most pressing in the emergency phase and it is also in this phase that the greatest logistic difficulties will be faced in providing basic care. Nevertheless, it is essential that a comprehensive assessment of the social, cultural, psychological and psychiatric aspects of any identified case is made to ensure that problems that are situational and contextually understandable are not labeled as severe mental illness and vice versa– the best safeguard being the involvement of a multidisciplinary team with a high level of cultural awareness. The balance of contributing factors to overall risk can vary – someone who is severely psychotic may be containable if living in an intact family structure whereas a person with an extreme grief reaction may be vulnerable if there is no family or kinship ties available to provide support. Where mental illness is present, interventions usual need to be multi-faceted with input from several sectors: mental health, social and welfare services, amongst others. The range of potential treatments is wide, ranging from crisis management and brief psychological interventions for severe trauma reactions (Straker, 1987) to pharmacological treatment for psychosis and severe depression.

The defined survival risk group (Figure 2) constitutes a small subgroup within post-conflict populations – often claimed to be 1%, (Silove et al., 2000) but in the absence of any statistics, more likely to be larger than this given the social definition offered herein. The error that can be made is to conclude that the smallness of the group makes the problem unimportant. In reality, the opposite inference should be drawn: affected persons often place not only themselves at risk but also the family and the wider community, hence creating a multiplier effect of threat (Figure 2); attempts to contain them can pre-occupy the time of aid workers and community leaders; failure to assist them erodes the already sensitive fabric of communities attempting to reconstitute themselves; short-term interventions can make a substantial impact; the circumscribed numbers needing urgent attention makes it feasible to mount small, cost-effective intervention programs with a clearly defined purpose; and the human rights risk faced by these persons means that attention to their plight falls clearly within the mandate of humanitarian relief efforts.

As indicated earlier, the larger group with psychological reactions to threat who are not immediately at survival risk pose a more complex problem in the emergency and immediate post-conflict setting – many will recover spontaneously as a state of safety and security returns, and as yet, the evidence remains equivocal whether individual or population-based interventions aimed at the prevention of long-term PTSD indeed effective (Raphael, 2000).

Figure 2. A stratified perspective on mental health needs of post-conflict settings

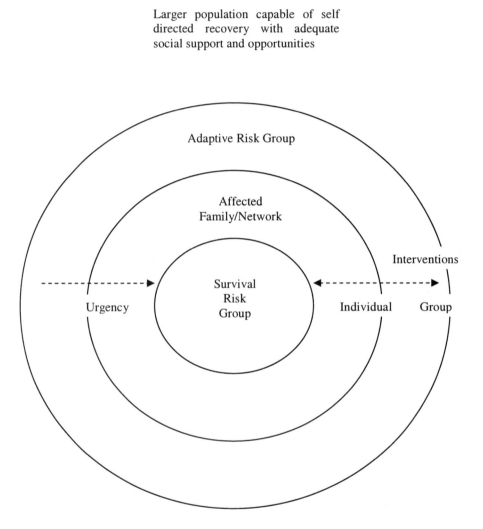

Larger population capable of self directed recovery with adequate social support and opportunities

Adaptive Risk Group

Affected Family/Network

Interventions

Survival Risk Group

Urgency   Individual   Group

Over time, a small percentage of the population is likely to manifest severe, ongoing trauma reactions that are disabling and which prevent adaptation – these persons warrant psychological attention as the emergency phase merges into the phase of recovery and reconstruction. Mental health services will also then become more stabilized and the approach to dealing with psychiatric needs will begin to approximate those that pertain in other developing countries.

3.2. The Attachment System

Similar considerations may be applied to the other survival and adaptive systems outlined in Figure 1. Unlike the "safety" system, the focus in the remaining systems tends to be on adaptation although reactions in a few may impair survival capacity. One of the key disruptions caused by mass violence and displacement is the impact of such events on the survivor's interpersonal bonds. Separations and losses often are multiple and include actual and symbolic losses. Acute grief is a natural and normative response to such events. Social interventions both in the emergency phase and beyond are the key to repairing ruptured bonds – where possible, families need to be traced and united, and it is essential to confirm the fate of those who are missing. One focus of social programs may be to assist in re-establishing culture-specific mourning rituals and to ensure that they are available to the population at large.

Exposure to loss *per se*, a common occurrence in situations of mass violence, does not mean that all affected persons need assistance, either in the emergency or in the reconstruction phases. Most people adapt and for some, the threats to bonds can lead to positive if painful adaptations. Survivors may learn to cherish family bonds in a deeper way than before, and priorities may be re-ordered so that great energy is directed to nurturing the young and to re-establishing and fostering kinship and community ties.

In a minority, grief reactions can be extreme in the acute phase, warranting crisis intervention (Raphael, 2000), and hence contributing to the subpopulation of persons defined as the high-risk group. In some, a form of chronic traumatic grief and depression may supervene (Prigerson et al., 1997; Horowitz et al., 1997; Raphael & Martinek, 1997). Hence, selective cases may warrant individual mental health interventions at a later stage in the social recovery process.

3.3. The Justice System

The human rights perspective is fundamental to understanding the role of social and psychological interventions in post-conflict societies. Torture, politically motivated sexual abuse, and internment in concentration camps, may constitute threats to life and safety but also exert their impact by dehumanizing, humiliating and degrading (Silove, 1996). When trapped in environments such as political prisons or concentration camps, inmates may be compelled to act in ways that ordinarily would be reprehensible to them and survival may be possible only by sacrificing or exploiting others. Forced betrayal, denunciation, and complicity commonly occur, with victims often being obliged to make impossible choices amongst alternatives that are equally reprehensible.

Subsequent events may compound the sense of injustice engendered by torture, rape, and acts of genocide. For example, survivors may find themselves living in a post-war society that remains riven by factionalism, plagued by corruption, and devoid of effective systems of justice; displaced communities confined in refugee camps may experience further exploitation and arbitrary treatment; and asylum seekers may endure prolonged periods of insecurity living in societies that are hostile to their presence. Also, perpetrators may live with impunity in survivor societies, thus confronting victims daily with the inadequacies of available mechanisms for indicting those guilty of crimes against humanity.

In the emergency phase, the key intervention is the provision of protection for those at risk of further persecution or victimization – the core purpose of the United Nations

Convention on Refugees (1951). Social, legal, political and, at times, military actions are fundamental to achieving a context free of further abuses. In the longer term, social responses to mass injustice include the re-establishment of a criminal justice system, war crimes indictments and prosecutions, truth and reconciliation commissions, systems for compensation, and local rituals that exact punishment and/or encourage dignified forgiveness. These initiatives take time and can rarely be accomplished in the immediate post-conflict phase, although the foundations of such activities, such as obtaining testimony, may be commenced early in the process.

Acute responses to injustices include individual or group expressions of anger and frustration and it is important that such reactions are not labelled as deviant or expressions of mental illness. Mental health professionals may be asked to advise in dealing with these situations, for example, in devising a humane approach to dealing with group protests or riots in crowded refugee camps – in most instances, issues relating to real or perceived injustices can be identified as root causes.

In the longer term, some survivors of persecution may adapt to their experiences by becoming fierce defenders of justice and human rights. Their personal experiences, however painful, may deepen their capacity for compassion for the suffering of others. For a minority, the extreme sense of injustice provoked by their ill-treatment may lead to adaptive difficulties, especially related to the control and expression of anger (Gorst-Unsworth et al., 1993; Ochberg, 1993; Davenport, 1991; Silove, 1996). Various formulations have been offered to classify such reactions (Beltran & Silove, 1999) but there is no unanimity on this issue. It is noteworthy that, unlike other affective reactions (depression, anxiety), there are no primary anger syndromes in conventional psychiatric typologies. In the western literature, it is usually assumed that anger is one manifestation (and hence subsumed by) disorders such as PTSD, depression or grief. Further work is needed therefore to investigate the phenomenology of chronic, disabling anger seen in a minority of survivors of human rights violations. In a selective number of cases in which future adaptation is grossly impaired, strategies for the treatment of such individuals may be warranted.

3.4. The Existential-Meaning System

Exposure to inexplicable evil and cruelty can shake the foundations of the survivor's faith in the beneficence of life and humankind. The extreme violation of torture often leaves survivors with existential preoccupations in which they strive, often unsuccess-fully, to find a coherent reason for the abuses they have suffered. They and their communities face a crisis of trust, faith, and meaning that may intensify feelings of alien-ation and emotional isolation (Gorst-Unsworth et al., 1993).

Such feelings may shape behaviors and attitudes in the immediate post-conflict phase and for years thereafter. Communities may find it difficult to trust external agencies offering assistance and it may take time for an ethos of participation and partnership to be established. Suspicion of authorities and of outsiders following years of oppression may be attributed erroneously to the national character or the culture of the local population, especially if outsiders are not familiar with the history of the conflict. Understanding these issues is vital to ensure an effective engagement of humanitarian aid workers and their organizations with the indigenous group, and mental health professionals may have special insights in advising other agencies about such matters.

At the same time, mental health professionals should be careful not to claim any special expertise in finding immediate solutions to these complex issues. Overcoming mistrust and feelings of alienation is a gradual process and depends largely on progress made in the social environment. The re-establishment of religious institutions and the rediscovery of spiritual faith may help to mitigate feelings of alienation as may engagement in meaningful political activities and the development of a sense of common purpose in the society as a whole. Although not usually the primary reason for mental health intervention, existential issues invariably form part of the complex array of problems professionals face in offering interventions for survivors in the longer term (Kinzie and Boehlein, 1993).

3.5. The Identity/Role System

One of the key aims of an oppressive regime is to undermine the person's sense of identity, agency and control. Indoctrination, propaganda, ostracism and isolation are all techniques that oppressive regimes use to undermine cohesion and identity in individual dissidents as well as in entire communities. Physical injury, mutilation and subsequent disability add to alterations in self-concept and the sense of identity of survivors. Being divested of one's social position, role, possessions and employment not only represent a loss and a violation, but also a potent threat to one's feelings of empowerment, efficacy, and individuality. Forced displacement, loss of culture and land, and resettlement in an alien and, at times, forbidding environment, further challenge the person's identity and capacity to control his/her destiny.

Again, the key interventions for the generality of the population are social, cultural, political and economic. The availability of work (Beiser et al., 1993) and other meaningful activities is critical to the goal of recreating a sense of purpose and identity for most persons. Participating in the restoration of a society's heritage and culture and the development of new structures that offer foster justice and communal participation helps to restore a sense of collective identity.

Maladaptive social responses in a minority may include extreme passivity and an excessive abnegation of roles. Some of these features have been codified in the still controversial ICD-10 category of 'Enduring Personality Change After Catastrophic Events' (Beltran & Silove, 2000). In all interventions, mental health professionals invariably focus on strengthening roles and the sense of identity, whether at the community or individual level, and they often work in concert with social, cultural, rehabilitation and employment agencies in order to approach the problem in a multidisciplinary manner.

4. CONCLUSIONS

The model proposed herein attempts to address some of the contentious issues that continue to bedevil the field of mental health in post-conflict situations. The central tasks of maximizing survival capacity in the emergency phase and setting the groundwork for communal adaptation in the reconstruction phase form the anchor points of the model. Recognition is given to the scarcity of resources available for mental health initiatives in such settings, and the importance of determining the urgency of needs based on the likelihood of survival and adaptive failures. Identifying the group at greatest survival risk is a priority in the acute phase of a humanitarian crisis and providing emergency care is an achievable goal. Some of those in greatest need will manifest acute trauma related reactions but the majority with traumatic symptoms will recover spontaneously. In contrast, predicting those at risk of adaptive failures in the medium to long-term is a more complex undertaking. Less certain is the effectiveness of population-based psychological interventions aimed at preventing the long-term mental consequences of trauma exposure. At the same time, a small group with disabling trauma reactions will emerge over time and they warrant special attention. There are strong arguments in support of pursuing concrete social strategies that lay the groundwork to allow the community to mobilize its own adaptive systems and thereby engage in the process of assuming responsibility for its own future.

Many challenges stand in the way of implementing these principles in a coherent fashion. As indicated earlier, elements of the emergency and reconstruction phase often intermingle and it is often necessary to pursue both elements simultaneously. Fragmentation in efforts, logistic and funding constraints, and a myriad of other obstacles always challenge the efforts of relief and development operations. The mental health enterprise faces particular credibility issues and its claim to legitimate participation is always at risk of being weakened by the contradictory claims of its proponents. Although complete consensus on priorities in mental health remains an aspiration rather than a reality, there is potential for achieving some common ground amongst competing models – the present contribution attempts to make some progress in that direction.

REFERENCES

Agger, I., Vuk, S., & Mimica, J. (1995) *Theory and Practice of Psychosocial Projects under War Conditions in Bosnia-Herzegovina and Croatia.* Zagreb: ECHO/ECTF.

Allden, K., Poole, C., Chantavanich, S., Ohmar, K., Aung, N.N. & Millica, R.F. (1996) Burmese political dissidents in Thailand: trauma and survival among young adults in exile. *American Journal of Public Health 86,*1561-1569.

Basoglu, M., Paker, M. & Paker, O. et al. (1994) Psychological effects of torture: A comparison of tortured with non-tortured political activists in Turkey. *American Journal of Psychiatry 151,*76-81.

Beiser, M., Johnson, P. J. & Turner, R. J. (1993) Unemployment, underemployment and depressive affect among South East Asian refugees. *Psychological Medicine 23,*731-743.

Beltran, R.O., & Silove, D. (1999) Expert opinions about the ICD-10 category 'Enduring Personality Change after Catastrophic Experience (EPCACE)'. *Comprehensive Psychiatry 40,* 1-9.

Bowlby, J. (1969) Attachment and Loss, *Attachment,* Vol.1. London: Penguin Books.

Cuny, F.C. (1983) *Disasters and development.* Oxford: Oxford University Press, 1-278.

Davenport, D. S. (1991) The functions of anger and forgiveness: guidelines for psychotherapy with victims. *Psychotherapy 28,*140-144.

Davies, A.P. (1996) Targeting the vulnerable in emergency situations: who is vulnerable? *The Lancet 348,* 868-871.

De Vries, F. (1998) To make a drama out of a trauma is fully justified. *Lancet 351,*1579-1580.

Eitinger, L. & Strom, A. (1973) *Mortality and Morbidity after Excessive Stress.* New York: Humanities Press.

Fleming, M.P. & Difede, J. (1999) Effects of varying scoring rules of the Clinician Administered PTSD Scale (CAPS) for the diagnosis of PTSD after acute burn injury. *Journal of Traumatic Stress 12,* 541.

Green, B. (1996) Traumatic Stress and Disaster: Mental Health Effects and Factors Influencing Adaptation. In Mak F. & Nadelson C. (eds.), *International Review of Psychiatry,* 177-211.

Gorst-Unsworth, C. & Goldenberg, E. (1998) Psychological sequelae of torture and organised violence suffered by refugees in Iraq. Trauma-related factors compared with social factors in exile. *British Journal of Psychiatry 172,* 90-94.

Gorst-Unsworth, C., Van Velsen, C. & Turner, S. (1993) Prospective pilot study of survivors of torture and organised violence: examining the existential dilemma. *Journal of Nervous and Mental Disease 181,* 263-264.

Hargreaves, W., LeGoullon, M., Gaynor, J. et al. (1984) Defining the severely mentally disabled. *Evaluation and Program Planning 7,* 219-227.

Harrell-Bond, B.E. (1986) *Imposing aid: emergency assistance to refugees.* Oxford: Oxford University Press.

Horowitz, M. J., Siegal, B. Holen, A. et al. (1997) Diagnostic Criteria for Complicated Grief Disorder, *American Journal of Psychiatry 154,* 904-910.

Kessler, R.C., (2000) Posttraumatic stress disorder: the burden to the individual and to society. *Journal of Clinical Psychiatry 13,* 4-12.

Kessler, R.C., Sonnega, A., Bromet, E,. Hughes, M. & Nelson, C.B. (1995) Posttraumatic stress disorder in the National Comorbidity Survey. *Archives of General Psychiatry 52,* 1048-1060.

Kinzie, J. D. & Boehnlein, J. K. (1993) Psychotherapy of the victims of massive violence: counter-transference and ethical issues. *American Journal of Psychotherapy 7,* 90-102.

Kirmayer, L. (1989) Cultural variations in the response to psychiatric disorders and mental distress. *Social Science & Medicine 26,* 327-329.

Kleinman, A. (1987) Anthropology and psychiatry; the role of culture in cross-cultural research on illness. *British Journal of Psychiatry 151,* 447-454.

Kleinman, A. (1988) *Rethinking Psychiatry: From Cultural Category to Personal Experience.* New York: Free Press.

Malt, U. F., Schnyder, U. and Weisaeth, L. (1996) ICD-10 mental and behavioral consequences of traumatic stress. In F. L. Mak and C. C. Nadelson (eds.), *International Review of Psychiatry 2.* Washington: American Psychiatric Press, 151-176.

Meltzer, H., Gill, B., Petticrew, M. et al. (1995) *OPCS Surveys of psychiatric morbidity in Great Britain, Report 2. Physical Complaints. Service Use and treatment of adults with psychiatric disorders.* London: HSMO.

Middleton, N., O'Keefe, P. (1998) *Disaster and Development. The Politics of Humanitarian Aid.* London: Pluto Press, 1-185.

Minas, H. & Silove, D., (2001) Transcultural and Refugee Psychiatry. In Bloch, S., Singh., B. (eds.), *Foundations of Clinical Psychiatry.* Melbourne: Melbourne University Press, 475-490.

Modvig, J., Pagaduan-Lopez, J., Rodenburg, C. et al. (2000) Torture and trauma in post-conflict East Timor. *The Lancet 356,* 1763.

Mollica, R. & Caspi-Yavin, Y. (1992) Overview: the assessment and diagnosis of torture events and symptoms. In M. Basoglu (ed.), *Torture and its Consequences* Cambridge: Cambridge University Press, 253-274.

Mollica, R. F., Caspi-Yavin, Y., Bollini, P. et al. (1992) The Harvard Trauma Questionnaire: Validating a cross-cultural instrument for measuring torture, trauma, and posttraumatic stress disorder in Indo Chinese refugees. *The Journal of Nervous and Mental Disease 180*,111-116.

Mollica, R. F., Donelan, K. & Tor, S. et al. (1993) The effect of trauma and confinement on functional health and mental health status of Cambodians living in Thailand-Cambodia border camps. *Journal of the American Medical Association 270*, 581-586.

Mollica, R.F., McInnes, K. & Sarajlic, N. et al. (1999) Disability associated with psychiatric co-morbidity and health status in Bosnian refugees living in Croatia. *Journal of American Medical Association 282*, 433-439.

Mollica, R., (2000) Special Report: Waging a new kind of war. Invisible Wounds. *Scientific American* (June 2000), 36-39.

Ochberg, F. M. (1993) Posttraumatic therapy. In: J. P. Wilson and B. Raphael (eds.), *International Handbook of Traumatic Stress Syndromes*. New York: Plenum Press, 773-783.

Peters, L., Slade, T., Andrews, G. (1999) A comparison of ICD10 and DSM-IV criteria for posttraumatic stress disorder. *Journal of Traumatic Stress 12*, 335-343.

Pitman, R.K., Altman, B., Greenwald, E. et al. (1991) Psychiatric complications during flooding therapy for post-traumatic stress disorder. *Journal of Clinical Psychiatry, 52*,17-20.

Priebe, S. & Esmaili, S. (1997) Long-term mental sequelae of torture in Iran – who seeks treatment? *Journal of Nervous and Mental Disease 185*, 74-77.

Prigerson, H. G., Shear, M. K. & Frank, E. et al. (1997) Traumatic grief: A case of loss-induced trauma. *American Journal of Psychiatry, 154*,1003-1009.

Raphael, B. & Martinek, N. (1997) Assessing Traumatic bereavement and Posttraumatic Stress Disorder. In: J. P. Wilson & T. M. Keane (eds.), *Assessing Psychological Trauma and PTSD*. New York: The Guilford Press, 373-395.

Raphael, B., Meldrum, L., McFarlane, A. (1995) Does debriefing after psychological trauma work? *British Medical Journal 310*,1479-1480.

Raphael, B., Wilson, J.P., (eds.) (2000) *Psychological Debriefing Theory, Practice and Evidence*. Cambridge: Cambridge University Press.

Raphael, B., Wilson, J.P. (2000) Introduction and Overview: Key issues in the conceptualisation of debriefing. In Raphael, B., Wilson, J.P. (eds.), *Psychological Debriefing Theory, Practice and evidence*. Cambridge: Cambridge University Press, 1-17.

Reinke, W., Hopwood, I., Knippenberg, R. (1997) Sustainability of primary health care including immunizations in Bamako Initiative programs in West Africa: An assessment of 5 years' field experience in Benin and Guinea. *International Journal of Health Planning and Management 12*, S1-S3.

Shalev, A. (2000) Stress management and debriefing: historical concepts and present patterns. In Raphael, B., Wilson, J.P. (eds.), *Psychological Debriefing Theory, Practice and evidence*. Cambridge: Cambridge University Press, 17-32.

Sen, A. (1990) Food, economics, and entitlements In Dreze, J., Sen., A. (eds.), *The Political Economy of Hunger*. Vol. 1, *Entitlement and Well-Being*. Oxford: Clarendon Press, 34-52.

Sen, A. (1989) Development as capability expansion. In Griffin, K., Knight, J., (eds.), *Human development and the international development strategy for the 1990's*. London: Macmillan, 41-58.

Sen, A. (1999a) Introduction: Development as Freedom. In Sen, A. (ed.), *Development as Freedom*. New York: Random House Inc., 3-13.

Sen, A. (1999b) Culture and Human Rights. In Sen, A. (ed.), *Development as Freedom*. New York: Random House Inc., 227-248.

Shrestha, N. M., Sharma, B. & van Ommeren, M. et al. (1998) Impact of torture on refugees displaced within the developing world. *Journal of American Medical Association 280*, 443-448.

Silove D. (1995) Prevention of psychosocial disability in victims of persecution and social chaos. In: Raphael, B. & Burrows, G. (eds.), *Handbook of Studies on Preventive Psychiatry*. Amsterdam: Elsevier Science BV, 343-357.

Silove, D. (1996) Torture and refugee trauma: implications for nosology and treatment of posttraumatic syndromes. In Mak, F.L. & Nadelson, C.C. (eds.), *International Review of Psychiatry 2*,151-176. Wasgington: American Psychiatric Press, 211-232.

Silove, D. (1999) The psychosocial effects of torture, mass human rights violations and refugee trauma: Towards an integrated conceptual framework. *The Journal of Nervous and Mental Disease 187*, 200-207.

Silove, D. (2000a), A conceptual framework for mass trauma: implications for adaptation, intervention and debriefing, in: *Psychological Debriefing, Theory Practice and evidence*, Raphael B & Wilson J P. (eds.), Cambridge University Press, 337-351.

Silove, D. (2000b) Trauma and Forced Relocation. *Current Opinions in Psychiatry 13*, 231-236.

Silove, D., Ekblad, S., Mollica, R. (2000) The rights of the severely mentally ill in post-conflict societies. *The Lancet 355*, April 29, 1548-1549.

Silove, D., Sinnerbrink, I., Field, A. et al. (1997) Anxiety, depression and PTSD in asylum seekers: associations with pre-migration trauma and post-migration stressors. *British Journal of Psychiatry 170*, 351-357.

Silove, D., Tarn, R. & Bowles, R. et al. (1991) Psychosocial needs of torture survivors. *Australian and New Zealand Journal of Psychiatry, 25*, 481-490.

Sirleaf, E.J. (1993) From disaster to development. In: Cahill, K.M. (ed.), *A framework for survival. Health, human rights, and humanitarian assistance in conflicts and disasters.* New York: Harper Collins, 299-307.

Simpson, M. (1993) Traumatic Stress and the bruising of the soul: the effects of torture and coercive interrogation. In: J. Wilson & B. Raphael (eds.), *International Handbook of Traumatic Stress Syndromes.* New York: Plenum Press, 667-684.

Skylv, G. (1992) The physical sequelae of torture. In: M. Basoglu (ed.), *Torture and its Consequences.* Cambridge: Cambridge University Press, 38-55.

Somasundaram, D. J. & Sivayokan, S. (1994) War trauma in a civilian population. *British Journal of Psychiatry 165*, 524-527.

Steel, Z., Silove, D., Bird, K. et al. (1999) Pathways from war trauma to posttraumatic stress symptoms amongst Tamil asylum seekers, refugees and immigrants. *Journal of Traumatic Stress 12*, 421-435.

Straker, G. (1987) The continuous traumatic stress syndrome – The single therapeutic interview. *Psychology in Society 8*, 48-79.

Stubbs, P. & Soroya, B. (1996) War trauma, psycho-social projects and social development in Croatia. *Medicine, Conflict and Survival 12*, 303-314.

Summerfield, D. (1997a) Legacy of war: beyond "trauma" to the social fabric. *The Lancet 349*, 1568.

Summerfield, D. (1997b) South Africa: does a truth commission promote social reconciliation? *British Medical Journal, 315*, 1393.

Summerfield, D. (1999) A critique of seven assumptions behind psychological trauma programs in war-affected areas. *Social Science and Medicine 48*, 1449-1462.

Toole, M. J., Waldman, R.J. (1988) An analysis of mortality trends among refugee populations in Somalia, Sudan, and Thailand. *Bulletin of the World Health Organization 66*, 237-247.

Toole, M. J., Waldman, R. J. (1990) Prevention of excess mortality in refugee and displaced populations in developing countries *Journal of American Medical Association 263*, 3296-3302.

Van Damme, W. (1995) Do refugees belong in camps? Experiences from Goma and Guinea. *Lancet, 346*, 360-362.

Van Damme, W. (1998a) Food Aid. In: *Medical Assistance to Self-settled Refugees, Guinea, 1990-96. Studies in Health Services Organisation and Policy 11*, 63-98.

Van Damme, W. (1998b) Health services for refugees: between primary health care and emergency medical assistance. In: *Medical Assistance to Self-settled Refugees, Guinea, 1990-96. Studies in Health Services Organisation and Policy 11*, 139-194.

Waldron, S.R. (1987) Blaming the refugees. *Refugee Issues 3*, 1-19.

Zarin, D.A. & Earls, F. (1993) Diagnostic decision making in psychiatry. *American Journal of Psychiatry 150*, 197-206.

3. TRANSFORMING LOCAL AND GLOBAL DISCOURSES:
Reassessing the PTSD movement in Bosnia and Croatia

Paul Stubbs[1]

1. INTRODUCTION

The wars of the Yugoslav succession, beginning in 1991 and culminating in the still unresolved Kosovo crisis, have seen large-scale killings and forced population movement as explicit major war aims, often euphemistically referred to as 'ethnic cleansing'. In this chapter, the dreadful realities of the wars and their wider socio-political contexts are less directly the focus than the ways in which these realities were reproduced and connected in specific, more or less coherent, discourses. These discourses were embedded in particular movements, which constructed ways of addressing and understanding the consequences of the conflicts on particular affected populations, and, most importantly, thereby delineated particular kinds of responses to ameliorate these consequences. Above all, the paper attempts to unravel the ways in which forms of psychosocial assistance, primarily defined in terms of post-traumatic stress disorder (PTSD), came to attain an important position within emergency responses to refugees and displaced persons in Croatia and Bosnia-Herzegovina.

The text builds on arguments which, together with Baljit Soroya, and based on research undertaken in Croatia from October 1993, I have advanced elsewhere regarding the problematic aspects of the dominant psychosocial discourse, particularly in Croatia (Stubbs & Soroya, 1996; Soroya & Stubbs, 1998). It is a reassessment, however, written some three years after I last focused, directly, on questions of PTSD and is much more a contribution to a sociology of organizational and professional responses to war and forced migration, in which the discourse and movement is addressed much more directly and viewed as more fractured and contradictory than previously. In addition, and consequently, critiques themselves, of which I was a part, are themselves understood as

---

[1] Paul Stubbs, Institute of Economics, Zagreb, Croatia.

discourses and movements which may have had effects which were either unintended, problematic or both.

Perhaps even more importantly, the text is a reconceptualization of an emerging critical orthodoxy that sees the PTSD movement as a 'new form of humanitarian intervention' (Parker, 1996) in which Western understandings and approaches are imposed, by aid agencies, on unsuspecting non-western populations. Whilst this argument has its merits, it is too sketchy and all-encompassing an explanation, neglecting the active role of key individuals and agencies and, even more importantly, the difficulty of Western professional discourses attaining a dominant global position without some form of connection with more locally specific discourses and practices. A close attention to discourses and movements suggests that emancipatory forms of analysis and practice are more likely to be prefigured by an examination of complexity and contradictions than by a simplistic either/or approach, and in which crude dichotomies between global and local, and indeed, between Western and non-western forms, are seen to have only limited explanatory value.

The next section provides a more detailed exposition of the Who and What of the dominant PTSD movement in Bosnia-Herzegovina and Croatia, from its establishment in late 1992. The section also attempts, somewhat tentatively and speculatively, to address How and Why the movement attained the importance it did and, in particular, to look at its relationship to other discourses and movements. The third section of this paper addresses the critique of the PTSD movement and its demise, and suggests ways in which a more nuanced understanding of the discourse of which it was critical, could have led to some different emphases. A brief concluding section looks at other approaches to refugee mental health based more on anthropological understandings of exile experiences and, on this basis, draws some brief lessons from the case study of relevance to practice and research, and more importantly, to emerging connections between the two, in the future.

2. THE PTSD MOVEMENT: MEANINGS, MOBILIZATIONS, AND MODALITIES

> This unexpected European war ... is probably the first war ever where not only the body and the material needs but also the soul and the psychological needs of the traumatized has (sic) been taken seriously on *a large scale*. (Arcel, 1994, *emphasis in original.*)

This quote comes from a book of proceedings from a conference, held in Zagreb, in April 1994 on "Psychosocial Care of Traumatized Women and Children: need for new methods and aims?" and it is a clear statement of the innovative nature of the approach by one of its leading proponents. By the time of the conference, the psychosocial approach, dominated by a particular understanding of PTSD, framed such a wide range of interventions, from a variety of agencies in Bosnia and Croatia, as to be clearly identifiable as a movement. By this time, four key agencies, and five key individuals, were playing a key role in its amplification:

1. The European Community Task Force (ECTF) and its psychosocial consultants *Libby Arcel* and *Inger Agger*. The ECTF was established at the EU Summit in Birmingham in October 1992 as the implementing body of the EU aid agency ECHO. In addition to its more usual aid and logistical operations, and following the Warburton report on rapes of women in Bosnia, it added the aim 'to develop, improve and coordinate the contribution of the European Union in the psychosocial field' (Martinez-Espinez, 1994). As usual with ECHO, it did not work directly with governments but, rather, funded a wide range of projects in the psychosocial field, mostly led by member-state NGOs, in Bosnia and Croatia.

2. The World Health Organization (WHO) and its Mental Health Consultant *Soren Buus Jensen*. Within a broad 'rehabilitation of war victims project', Jensen headed a mental health unit concerned both "to protect the mental health of populations in 'Former Yugoslavia' and to prepare national mental health services for post-war development" (Jensen, 1994), which involved research, training and support primarily to governmental agencies and to local experts.

3. The United Nations Children's Fund (UNICEF) and its psychosocial Advisor *Rune Stuvland*. In parallel with WHO, UNICEF also focused on research, training, and project support, with a particular emphasis on children as victims of war, and with a wider range of initiatives including some work with local NGOs, again throughout 'Former Yugoslavia'.

4. The United Nations High Commissioner for Refugees (UNHCR) and its Regional Social Services Officer *Marcia Jacobs*. Perhaps less important in stressing PTSD than the other agencies, UNHCR was a major funder of NGO psychosocial projects working with refugees in Croatia and Bosnia. The main link is, however, through Jacobs' co-authoring of a core theory and practice text on 'what defines a psychosocial project' with two others in the movement (Agger, Jensen, and Jacobs, 1995), which they described as 'a truly collaborative effort'.

Designating these organizations and individuals as a 'movement' may be less accurate than seeing them as an epistemic community or a network of knowledge based experts. Certainly, there are strong epistemic and related links between four of the five, three being from Denmark, two of whom (Agger and Jensen) were, at the time, married to each other, and a fourth, Stuvland, from Norway so that a Scandinavian perspective is apparent, instantly, as dominant. All sought explicitly to link theory, research and practice and were very conscious, as the quote from Arcel demonstrates, of the pioneering nature of their intervention. The innovative organizational core, in many ways, for the group, is the ECTF, in terms of levels of funding, extent of dissemination of analysis, and the development of new approaches. ECTF as an implementing body of ECHO, itself at that time a relatively new humanitarian actor, can be considered in terms of its two key aspects - as a European and as an emergency aid agency, hence already, almost *a priori* as it were, tending to exclude any non European and developmental approaches.

Seeing ECTF as a key part of the way in which humanitarian intervention substituted for political intervention is only part of the story. At the onset of the refugee crisis in Bosnia, with large numbers of refugees arriving in Croatia, itself with large numbers of displaced persons, a major theme was the systematic rape of, primarily Bosnian Muslim women. It was on this basis, with Libby Arcel herself playing a leading role, that psychosocial support redefined in terms of 'vulnerable women and children', was added to ECTF's mandate. In other words, a politicized context helped to set up a relatively autonomous and explicitly depoliticized professional psychosocial field, more or less free to develop explanations, analyses, and projects, provided these did not impinge upon or threaten wider power relations or other aspects of the European Union's interventions.

2.1. The psychosocial Field

In retrospect, notwithstanding differences of emphasis, the psychosocial field was established on the basis of three core elements, which, in shorthand terms, can be labeled 'essentializing trauma'; talking up the numbers; and justifying intervention. All of these are, of course, highly problematic and, in other circumstances, would certainly be questioned by some or all of the individuals involved in establishing the field, aware as they surely were of an emerging general critical psychological literature. Taken together, they amount to a very questionable argument that PTSD is a relatively unproblematic diagnostic category; that large numbers of refugees and displaced persons in Croatia and Bosnia-Herzegovina suffer from it; and that massive psychological assistance, including from internationals, is required to treat it. It is as if, to establish such a field, and to convince a number of influential publics, a crude, and lowest common denominator approach had to be installed in the core before more nuanced understandings could be introduced. In some ways, this is a kind of classic moral entrepreneurship in which a 'moral panic' approach to a social problem frames a limited range of solutions. Each of the core elements, as strands in the discourse, can be noted briefly here.

2.1.1. Essentializing Trauma

Throughout the public presentations of the work of ECTF, there was an essentializing of the concept of PTSD as 'a set of symptoms which follow a trauma outside of the range of usual experience' and which contained a number of essential features. (Arcel, 1994) The term 'trauma' tends, therefore, to be used to describe an event or series of events, a symptom or series of symptoms, and a condition, so that, in a key elision, people become their symptoms and their experiences, and can be referred to, unproblematically, as 'traumatized children' (Stuvland, 1994) or, simply, 'the traumatized' (Agger, Jensen and Jacobs, 1995).

In the same literature, however, there are the beginnings of a much more nuanced approach, in terms of the importance of strengthening ' psychosocial protective factors' and decreasing ' psychosocial stressor factors' (Agger, Jensen & Jacobs, 1995) which should have opened the door to much more reflection on the broader social, political and cultural dimensions of lived experiences. This insight is never pursued, however, so that the essentialist perspective on trauma, delinked from any wider structures, retains a core position.

2.1.2. Talking Up the Numbers

A key text, referring to an unpublished WHO study co-authored by Jensen, suggested as early as late 1994 that 'more than 700,000 people in Bosnia-Herzegovina and Croatia ... suffer from severe psychic trauma' (Agger, Jensen & Jacobs, 1995), with Jensen, in an influential *New York Times* article in January 1995, quoted as stating that 'there is no doubt in my mind that post-traumatic stress is going to be the most important public health problem in the former Yugoslavia for a generation and beyond' (Kinzler, 1995). The WHO study, which I have not seen, appears to estimate these numbers on the basis of a series of statistical assumptions about the existence of severe trauma in peacetime and in war time conditions, including a figure of 20% of all refugees and displaced persons, which is not only, itself, questionable, but, of course, relies on what was, at the time, a rather questionable figure of forced migrant numbers (Spirer, 1995).

Preliminary data from 1974 people in one psychosocial project in Zagreb concluding that 'a great number of people ... had considerable losses, deep traumatic experiences and needed urgent social support' (Arcel, 1994) and from a screening of children in 28 schools in Croatia (Stuvland, 1994) are, perhaps, more valuable but also suffer from a number of methodological flaws and, above all, little validity as representative samples. Guesswork seems to have been more important in amplifying the nature of the problem as well as contributing to an illusion of planning, not least since most psychosocial projects were being implemented in the relative safety of Croatia and most suffering, even according to the assumptions of the WHO study, was in Bosnia where 78% of the affected population was said to be based, people who were receiving very little support (Agger, Jensen & Jacobs, 1995).

2.1.3. Justifying Intervention

The sentence quoted above about the large numbers suffering from severe psychic trauma ends with the words 'and need urgent and qualified assistance' (Agger, Jensen & Jacobs, 1995). Local professionals were estimated to be sufficient to meet less than 1% of the needs for psychosocial assistance of the traumatized, therefore, both international assistance, and a wider range of interventions including those by para-professionals and non-professionals, were seen as needed. In typical moral entrepreneurship, failing to act would have disastrous consequences for at least the next two generations, in terms of increases in alcohol and drug addictions, suicides, all kinds of violence (criminal and domestic) and psychiatric illness and, in addition, unresolved traumatic experiences are likely to ignite new hatred and new wars (ibid.).

The balance between international and local staff, and between professionals and non-professionals, tended to be discussed somewhat abstractly, if at all. The argument that local mental health professionals were likely, in significant numbers, to be traumatized themselves, so that internationals, as well as prioritizing training, should reserve their practical work for this group served, as Derek Summerfield has commented wryly, "to aggrandize the status, knowledge and indeed health of the foreign expert" (Summerfield, 1996). The crudity of the lack of any kind of social or cultural awareness amongst members of this epistemic community, perhaps best exemplified by Inger Agger's infamous phrase "when I arrived in the former Yugoslavia" (Agger, 1995), is also reflected in a number of telling phrases and articles which suggest that, in large part, their main point of contact was other international humanitarian aid workers, all of whose 'longing for Sarajevo' (Agger, 1995) was mediated through this framework more than any others.

3. LEGITIMATING CONNECTIONS

Given the problematic nature of all of these strands of the discourse, the success of the PTSD movement can be considered as less a product of its internal coherence and much more a result of a series of real or imagined connections with more progressive discourses, themes and movements which, in shorthand terms, I shall call gendered perspectives, human rights, and civil society.

3.1. Gendered Perspectives

In some ways, the relationship with gendered perspectives was unsurprising given the origins of the psychosocial field in EU investigations, including the Warburton Commission, into rape as a weapon of war in Bosnia-Herzegovina. Given this fact, it is the way in which the psychosocial discourse makes virtually no mention of the connection, which is rather more remarkable, substituting instead a notion of women and children as vulnerable groups. It is certainly true that the response to systematic gendered violence, particularly by women's groups in Zagreb, some of whom had their origins in proto-feminist movements of the 1980s, and some with more nationalist agendas, did see trauma as a major issue to be dealt with, as part of a wide range of humanitarian, counseling, support, and political interventions. Indeed, some of the theoretical impetus for this may well have come from Judith Herman's 'Trauma and Recovery' (Herman, 1992), making connections between domestic violence and political violence, and which circulated widely amongst activists and, indeed was translated into Croatian by the Zagreb based Women's Infoteka.

3.2. Human Rights

In some ways, the gender perspective fed into a wider 'human rights' framework, not least because of the emphases of Inger Agger, herself the author of 'The Blue Room' (Agger, 1994), a pioneering study of gender, human rights and testimony in Chile which was also, interestingly, translated by Women's Infoteka. Indeed, having suggested that "(the) overall purpose of psychosocial emergency assistance is to promote mental health *and human rights*" (Agger, Jensen & Jacobs, 1995, *my emphasis*), one would expect to find copious references to how this could be done. In fact, apart from vague references to the importance of memory in peace building, there is little elaboration of the importance of testimony in terms of the International Criminal Court and wider questions of justice. Again, it is as if the dominant psychosocial field would be stretched too far if human rights were to be anything more than a rhetorical device. However, simply by mentioning one of the dominant leitmotifs of 'global ideoscapes' (Appadurai, 1996), there is a sense in which a progressive intent, more imagined than real it must be said, is hinted at.

3.3. Civil Society

The space opened up in terms of civil society also contributed to the progressive appearance of some elements of the PTSD movement but this is far more complex, given the split between ECTF and, to an extent, UNHCR, which primarily funded NGO-led projects, and WHO and UNICEF which, by and large, promoted initiatives with the governmental sectors. Nevertheless, and notwithstanding the vacuity of notions of civil society which are "undertheorised, insufficiently concretized in terms of specific practices, and rarely subject to critical scrutiny" (Stubbs, 1996a), by promoting a wide range of NGO activities, ECTF's funding of the psychosocial field did expand the space open to innovative projects. Some of these were, indeed, led by, or at least involved, local groups, activists and movements, including those who framed interventions more in terms of gender-based and human rights approaches. Whether the psychosocial shape was bent to include some of these projects or vice versa remains disputable, but the space opened up in a society where there had been very limited civil initiatives before the war, and where the state tended to monopolize health and social services, certainly could, in itself, secure support from those wishing to see an expansion of non-governmental activities.

In some ways, what was much more important was the way in which NGO-led psychosocial projects, based on the assumptions of the PTSD movement, multiplied in 1993 and 1994 as more and more agencies, including many significant donors, tended to follow the trend. Particularly important in what can, perhaps, be termed the second wave of projects were those supported by USAID which included two multi-million dollar programs, one an 'Umbrella Grant for Trauma and Reunification' through the US NGO *The International Rescue Committee* (IRC), which became the biggest local NGO support program in Bosnia and Croatia, and the other through a partnership between Catholic Relief Services (CRS) and the Croatian *NGO The Society for Psychological Assistance* (SPA) to implement a large-scale program on 'Trauma Recovery Training'.

4. ASPECTS OF THE PSYCHOSOCIAL SHAPE

Clearly, the defining of the psychosocial shape in terms of the need for new local NGOs benefited Croatian, and to an extent, Bosnian, psychologists and psychiatrists who became very much 'flavor of the month' - some forming their own NGOs, others involved in a range of supervisory, sessional, and consultancy work. In large part, of course, their market-value rose in response to the obvious critique of the failure of international organizations to understand refugees' language and culture and the importance of working with local professionals. There developed, in fact, a very complex relationship between international and local professionals, which has to be seen in the context of the history of the mental health training and practice infrastructure in Croatia and Bosnia before the war. This was very well developed with good connections with the international mental health community.

Within this local infrastructure, very diverse approaches to mental health tended to co-exist alongside each other, with less explicit antagonism than might be found in Western Europe, for example. A generally over-empiricist and labeling medical model, therefore, rested alongside some heavily Vienna-influenced psychoanalysis and an emerging discourse, certainly in Slovenia and parts of Croatia, in the 1980s, of anti-psychiatry, gestalt and other celebrations of self-awareness and identity which, in a dominant political framework which was perhaps over social in its orientation, could attain quite a radical import, even if they rarely impacted on day-to-day professional practice. Sometimes, individuals combined these diverse approaches and, when psychosocial work predominated so that all kinds of training courses were being offered, it was not unusual to see different, and from a Western gaze incompatible, approaches, being implemented together within the same project. I have argued elsewhere that, in fact, this flexibility, rather than any newly invented strategy, contributed to the ability to say different things to different audiences, thereby strengthening the discourse and movement rather than weakening it (Stubbs, 1997).

In addition, as already noted, an apparent tension within the movement was the fact that ECTF largely worked with NGOs and some other agencies, particularly WHO and UNICEF, worked with governmental agencies and academics, engaging much more with the existing mental health system. Indeed, to one critic of privatized, unregulated and multi-mandated NGO-led projectization, UNICEF's remarkable psychosocial program was seen as "a prototype for a cross-line institutional support and adaptation policy" (Duffield, 1994). In reality, this supported a psychological elite, particularly in Croatia, whose clinical approaches to PTSD tended to be reinforced rather than challenged. In any case, the categories of governmental, research and NGO provision tended to become blurred somewhat with members of this elite skilled in being involved in a wide range of initiatives. Even more importantly, despite Duffield's assertions, it was primarily in Croatia that this work was undertaken, so that the effects on Bosnian services, still at the time in war conditions, was only limited. Indeed, the ways in which the crisis allowed this local, though internationally connected, elite, to join the ranks of a global elite and, even now, to claim competence as the best placed to work with Kosovan refugees in Macedonia and Albania, is particularly instructive.

Overall, the effects of the emphasis on psychosocial approaches was much less to open up the field to a wider range of perspectives than to reinforce traditional hierarchies, between academics and practitioners, between professionals and non-professionals, between psychologists and members of other disciplines, and indeed between Croatia and Bosnia, and urban and rural areas within these countries. The extended amplification of these hierarchies further marginalized any attention, above and beyond rhetoric, to user involvement, community-based services, and that over-used term empowerment. Indeed, as the PTSD movement began to be critiqued, it was the work of NGOs, largely unsustainable because of their reliance on emergency foreign funding, which contracted, leaving the field to be dominated even more by the core, now closer to mainstream government-controlled services, in which prestigious projects, based on clinical, medicalizing, and pathologizing approaches, came to dominate.

5. CRITICAL PERSPECTIVES REASSESSED

It is very difficult, from the perspective of someone involved from the inside in opposing the PTSD movement, to assess what the impact of the critique was. It cannot be disputed, however, that by mid-1996, there was much less emphasis, certainly within priorities for funding of NGOs, on projects connected with 'trauma' questions. In part, this may have been a rational response to changing circumstances and needs, and to initial evaluations which tended, at best, to be inconclusive about the value of the most costly, expert-led, approaches. In some ways, in the post-Dayton situation of Bosnia-Herzegovina, questions of refugee return and of democratization became more pressing, and with other, newly formed, epistemic communities showing almost no interest in trauma questions - the limited impact which Inger Agger had when she moved to the OSCE in Bosnia is, perhaps, an indication of this. In addition, in Croatia, issues of the reintegration of Eastern Slavonia, of refugee return, and of support for a more balanced third sector also took precedence in the context, in any case, of declining international financial support.

Nevertheless, in the trend-based world of humanitarian aid and development, in which priorities are developed and sustained according to crude 'sound bites' as much as rational planning, the critique probably was important in challenging what had been up to that point, a more or less unshakeable belief in the psychosocial approach. Two anecdotes are, perhaps, relevant here. As early as the middle of 1995, I was approached by Jadranka Mimica, a Croatian psychologist working as assistant to Inger Agger in ECTF, who had been asked by ECTF in Brussels, to explore community development approaches. Finding common ground, we expanded our analysis in a text published in the *Community Development Journal* which stated that, in Croatia, 'the psycho- has dominated at the expense of the social' (Mimica & Stubbs, 1996; 286) and outlining a developmental agenda in which changes in communities not just in individuals could be promoted. Whilst it is hard to be certain, this perhaps signified, at least, a crack in the support for the psychosocial approach within the EU.

In addition, in June 1996, I was asked to speak at the Third Anniversary meeting of the IRC Umbrella Grant. My text, translated into Croatian, was published soon afterwards in the political weekly *Arkzin* where I again criticised "an over emphasis on so-called psychosocial programs heavily reliant on professional, labour intensive, and expensive psychological approaches to trauma, and reinforcing the cult of the expert, at the expense of much broader based social and community development approaches", going on to suggest "that the supposed emphases of some of these projects on self-help, empowerment, and such like, is little more than a smoke screen meant to hide the essentially pathologizing and hierarchical nature of service provision" (Stubbs, 1996b). Perhaps even more significantly, a short time later, a proposal which I had helped a local NGO to develop, for a community development project in a deprived area of Zagreb serving a socially excluded Roma population alongside refugees and an ageing and impoverished local community, which purposefully never mentioned psychosocial or trauma, was funded by the IRC Umbrella Grant. It was also praised as a prototype for the future at the same time, indeed, as the trauma element of the Umbrella Grant was dropped from its name.

In some ways, this was the culmination of over two years of pressure based on research, activism and practice in Croatia, in which I had advocated for social and community development frameworks which, in the midst of the dominance of psychosocial approaches, had seemed to be largely absent in Croatia. Collaborating closely at the time with Nina Pečnik, a founder of the grassroots NGO *Suncokret* and also a psychologist and Lecturer in Social Work at the University of Zagreb, we had drawn a division between three discourses:

Figure 1. Contrasting Features of Humanitarian Aid, psychosocial Projects, and Development Projects (Pečnik & Stubbs, 1995).

HUMANITARIAN AID	PSYCHOSOCIAL PROJECTS	DEVELOPMENTAL PROJECTS
Dependency	Expert	Flexible
Patronizing	Pathologizing	Empowering
Demeaning	Medicalizing	Engaged/Social Movement
Distorting of National	Distanced	Community
Economy	Professionalizing	Based/Localised
Needs of Donors Not	Inflexible	Integrating
Recipients	Prestigious For Workers	Transformative
Divisive	Not Users	Links/Connects Different
Disrespectful	Needs Defined by Experts	Levels
Emergency	Not Communities	Human Rights
Undermining Local	Disconnected from	Develops Skills
Communities	Community Needs	Democratic
Distributive Effects - ?	Self-Maintaining	Civil Society
Reinforcing Inequalities	Disempowering	Action Research
Unaccountable	Labeling e.g. PTSD	Long-term Planning
Self-Maintaining Business	Creates Elite	
Part of a War	Foreign Experts -	
Game/Reproduces War	Unaccountable	
Disempowering	Local Experts –	
Unjust	Accelerated Promotion and	
Fosters Mistrust	Salary	
Prevents Local Solidarity	Self-Fulfilling Evaluation -	
Actions	Narrow; Quantitative	
	Uncoordinated	
	Temporary	
	Duplicating	

Our work was, certainly, sustained by a series of international connections that suggested that we were not alone in being profoundly suspicious of the PTSD movement and had, perhaps, even underestimated its increasing global impact. I first became aware of Derek Summerfield's work, for example, during a visit to Belgrade in November 1994 where a worker with Oxfam which, astonishingly given its own social development profile, had initially prioritized work on trauma, gave me an unpublished text which had been crucial, for her, in questioning this emphasis. Later, Summerfield was instrumental in ensuring that a core critical text, co-written with Baljit Soroya, and which had circulated widely in the region, was finally published after having been rejected by another journal on the basis of criticisms from two referees both involved in the PTSD movement (Stubbs & Soroya, 1996). At the same time, he himself published a highly influential article, which used some of the same material in mounting a far more rigorous critique of psychosocial projects (Summerfield, 1996). Also influential was David Ingleby, first encountered through my brief subscription to an e-mail discussion group on post-traumatic stress, and who invited me to a conference on "health care for migrants and refugees" (Balledux & de Mare, 1995) where, again, a wider range of critical perspectives were elaborated.

In retrospect, then, the' critique of the PTSD movement in Croatia and Bosnia-Herzegovina moved, rather quickly, from the margins to the mainstream, in which it has now become something of an orthodoxy to state that PTSD is a highly disputed category, that estimates of numbers affected, and assumptions of the necessity of treatment, are problematic, and that "the ways in which people express and embody and give meaning to ... distress is largely dependent on context - social, cultural, political and economic" (Boyden & Gibbs, 1997). What had seemed like a very difficult target turned out not to be so at all, and to be so discredited that it has now become very difficult to get any international funding, certainly in Croatia, for innovative therapeutic work even though distress and longer-term consequences can be demonstrated. In some ways this is an argument that the critique was simply too all embracing and unfocused, based on the assumption of separate discourses and, of course, on the progressive nature of social and community development.

Rereading the texts for this paper, I am struck by how little they are focused concretely on the complexities of local and global discourses, much less on the differences between discourses, individual agents, and practices within particular projects. Whilst stating that the intention is not to deny suffering and distress but, rather to demonstrate the ways in which people are reduced to cases, expressions of hurt to symptoms, and processes of healing to treatment, there is a cumulative tendency to throw the baby out with the bathwater, and to argue for a complete rejection of one approach in favour of another. There is little real analysis of the complexities of diverse refugee experiences and responses, between those from Croatia compared with those from Bosnia, between urban and rural populations, between different ethno-religious and other identity-based groupings, and so on.

There is also no real confrontation with the specific nature of the atrocities which came to be termed ethnic cleansing, much less any call for more research on this. Perhaps unsurprisingly in the context of the period, there is little attempt to understand the How and Why of the psychosocial approach, to treat it as a complex set of ideas and practices, nor to engage with more progressive approaches from within. A number of initiatives which sought to combine trauma healing with peace building, for example, are conveniently ignored. Above all, the existence of different global and local constituencies, and the possibility of linking critical mental health perspectives within post-Yugoslav countries with those outside, was not really engaged with.

With the benefit of hindsight, of course, social development discourses proved to be no less problematic and, on numerous occasions, equally divorced from social, political and cultural realities. Above all, a naive faith in grassroots approaches resulted in almost no engagement with the project planning process and a refusal to take seriously the question 'if you had these funds, what would you do?' In short, an opportunity to break down a number of boundaries which obviously were problematic in terms of services for refugees in distress: between disciplines; between theory, research and practice; and between different knowledges-in-use from different global and local contexts, was missed.

6. CONCLUSIONS: REFUGEE MENTAL HEALTH OR AN ANTHROPOLOGY OF EXILE?

In some ways, my current interest is in seeking to refocus a connection between what might be termed refugee mental health questions, which have, of course taken on a more critical edge recently, and an anthropology of exile which starts with forced migrants' lived experiences but which can and should, seek to extend its methods to explore inter-actions with so-called helpers. Both, in their different ways, are increasingly concerned with complex concepts of 'cultures', 'identities', and forms of 'belongings' and 'losses' and, clearly, in terms of policy and practice development, there are many important benefits likely to come from cross-fertilization between the two approaches. Whilst Parker, one of the first to argue for this connection, is right to warn of the dangers of social anthropologists' 'culturalizing violence' (Parker, 1996), recent attempts to develop anthropological understandings of the 'global production of locality' (Appadurai, 1996) and of diverse kinds of 'travel encounters' (Clifford, 1997) are signposts towards a very different conceptual framework.

A collection of texts from a conference on War, Exile, Everyday Life, organized by young anthropologists from the Institute of Ethnology and Folklore Research in Zagreb (Jambrešić Kirin & Povrzanović, 1996) is a clear example of the possibilities here, and, elsewhere, Malkki's work on Rwanda (1995), is also highly instructive. In turning 'war and exile ... into domains of anthropological scrutiny' (Povrzanović & Jambrešić Kirin, 1996), producing a 'multivoiced ethnography of war' (Jambrešić Kirin, 1999), and combining 'critical abilities', 'emotional commitment', 'moral indignation' and 'political analysis' (Povrzanović & Jambrešić Kirin, 1996), the approach is suggestive of a new set of research questions, which may help to reorient critical perspectives on refugee mental health.

In lieu of conclusions, then, I want to state what seem to me to be some of the most pertinent questions for debate and discussion:

1. How can ethnographic understandings of war and exile as diverse processes and meanings influence what appear to be short-term, and quite narrow, agency-led psychosocial frameworks?

2. What do the testimonies of refugees tell us of their encounters with diverse help-ers and how might these be used to reorient policy and practice?

3. What processes may be at work in the ascription and achievement of certain labels, including that of trauma, amongst diverse refugee communities, and how do these labels affect roles, status, and access to resources?

4. In the encounter between project communities and refugee communities, who play the roles of intermediaries and interpreters, and how important are these in terms of processes and outcomes?

5. What factors in the response of diverse local communities to diverse refugee communities promote integration and healing? How do wider policy contexts affect these processes?

Whilst more research is, of course, needed, perhaps of equivalent value will be a re-examination of existing material, and support for testimony to be seen as an important part of the response to refugee emergencies, not only in the name of justice, but also healing. Above all, I am arguing that what Peter Loizos has termed 'allocation-words' (Loizos, 1996), which I would reframe somewhat as allocation processes, including the labels from within refugee mental health, are relevant directly to breaking down the split between 'a post-modern ethnography of fracture, disjunction, experience of suffering, and resistance' (Loizos, 1996) and 'socially worthwhile collaboration with planners and policy makers' (Loizos, 1996). These connections will not appeal to all and, indeed, too close a rapprochement is less likely to promote new perspectives, much less those which may be sustainable and genuinely progressive and in the interests of diverse refugee communities, than attempts to debate and discuss across these divisions.

REFERENCES

Agger, I. (1994) *The Blue Room: Trauma and testimony among refugee women - a psychosocial exploration.* London: Zed Books.

Agger, I. (1995) A longing for Sarajevo: understanding the trauma of humanitarian aid workers. In: Agger, I. (ed.), *Theory and practice of psychosocial projects under war conditions.* Zagreb: ECTF, 27-33.

Agger, I., Jensen, S., & Jacobs, M. (1995) Under War Conditions: what defines a psychosocial project?, In: Agger, I. (ed.), *Theory and practice of psychosocial projects under war conditions. Zagreb:* ECTF, 11-26.

Appadurai, A. (1996) *Modernity at Large: Cultural Dimensions of Globalization.* Minnesota: University of Minnesota Press.

Arcel, L. (1994) War victims, trauma and psychosocial care. In: Arcel, L. (ed.), *War Victims, Trauma and Psychosocial Care.* Zagreb: ECTF, 11-22.

Balledux, M. & de Mare, J. (eds.) (1995) *Ouder- en Kindzorg voor migranten en vluchtelingen* (Child Health Care for Migrants and Refugees). Assen: Van Gorcum.

Boyden, J. & Gibbs, S. (1997) *Children of War: responses to psychosocial distress in Cambodia.* Geneva: UNRISD.

Clifford, J. (1997) *Routes: travel and translation in the late twentieth century.* Cambridge: Harvard University Press.

Duffield, M. (1994) *Complex Political Emergencies: an exploratory report for UNICEF.* Mimeo, University of Birmingham.

Herman, J. (1992) *Trauma and Recovery.* New York: Basic Books.

Jambrešić Kirin, R. (1999) Personal Narratives on War: a challenge to women's essays and ethnography in Croatia. *Estudos de literatura oral 5,* 73-98.

Jambrešić Kirin, R. & Povrzanović, M., eds. (1996) *War, Exile, Everyday Life: Cultural perspectives.* Zagreb: IEF.

Jensen, S. (1994) Psychosocial stresses and protective factors in families under war conditions and peace building in former Yugoslavia. In Arcel, L. (ed.), *War Victims, Trauma and Psychosocial Care.* Zagreb: ECTF, 72-79.

Kinzler, S. (1995) In Croatia, minds scarred by war. *New York Times,* 9 January.

Loizos, P. (1996) Perspective from an earlier war. In Jambrešić Kirin, R. & Povrzanović, M. (eds.), *War, Exile, Everyday Life: Cultural perspectives.* Zagreb: IEF, 293-301.

Malkki, L. (1995) *Purity and Exile: Violence, memory and national cosmology.* Chicago: University Press.

Martinez-Espinez, F. (1994) Opening Speech. In Arcel, L. (ed.), *War Victims, Trauma and Psychosocial Care.* Zagreb: ECTF.

Mimica, J. & Stubbs, P. (1996) Between Relief and Development: Theories, practice and evaluation of psychosocial projects in Croatia. *Community Development Journal 31,* 281-290.

Parker, M. (1996) The Mental Health of War-damaged Populations. *IDS Bulletin 27,* 77-85.

Pečnik, N. & Stubbs, P. (1995) Croatia: from dependency to development? *Rural Extension Bulletin 8,* 35-39.

Povrzanović, M. & Jambrešić Kirin, R. (1996) Negotiating Identities? The voice of refugees between experience and representation. In Jambrešić Kirin, R. & Povrzanović, M. (eds.), *War, Exile, Everyday Life: Cultural perspectives*. Zagreb: IEF, 3-19.

Soroya, B. & Stubbs, P. (1998) Ethnicity, forced migration and psychosocial work in Croatia. *Medicine, Conflict and Survival 14*, 303-313.

Summerfield, D. (1996) The Impact of war and atrocity on civilian populations: basic principles for NGO interventions and a critique of trauma projects. *ODI Relief and Rehabilitation Network Paper 14*. London: ODI.

Spirer, L. (1995) Report from the Hague, December 8-10, 1994, for American Statistical Association Committee for Human Rights and Freedom Newsletter. http://www.virtualschool.edu/mon/news/UnWarTribunal

Stubbs, P. (1996a) Nationalisms, Globalization and Civil Society in Croatia and Slovenia. *Research in Social Movements, Conflicts and Change 19*, 1-26. http://www.stakes.fi/gaspp/ps_cv.htm

Stubbs, P. (1996b) NGO Development in Croatia: definitions and dilemmas (Croatian language version), *ArkZin*, 69, July.

Stubbs, P. (1997) NGO work with forced migrants in Croatia: lineages of a global middle class? *International Peacekeeping 4*, 50-60.

Stubbs, P. & Soroya, B. (1996) War trauma, psychosocial projects and social development in Croatia. *Medicine, Conflict and Survival 12*, 303-314.

Stuvland, R. (1994) School-age children affected by war: the UNICEF programme in former Yugoslavia. In Arcel, L. (ed.), *War Victims, Trauma and Psychosocial Care*. Zagreb: ECTF, 111-126.

4. TRAUMATIC STRESS IN CONTEXT
A study of unaccompanied minors
from Southern Sudan

Olle Jeppsson and Anders Hjern[1]

In 1986 tens of thousands of young boys with a traditional upbringing in the Dinka tribe escaped from the terror of civil war in southern Sudan into refuge in Ethiopia. In 1991 they were forced to move on, this time through southern Sudan into northern Kenya. In this article we present some experiences gained from relief work with this group during 1986-1994. We will summarize earlier reports and present findings from an interview study made in 1994, with the aim of contrasting the Western medical model of traumatic stress with the particular political and cultural context of the Dinkas of southern Sudan.

1. SOUTHERN SUDAN

The conflict between southern and northern Sudan can be traced back thousands of years. The current conflict between the Islamic, Arabic north and the African, animist/Christian south started around 600 AD with the intrusion of Arabic tribes. It was

[1] Olle Jeppsson, Department of Pediatrics, Huddinge University Hospital, Karolinska Institutet, Stockholm, Sweden; Anders Hjern, National Board of Health and Welfare, Center for Epidemiology, Stockholm, Sweden.

strengthened by the slave trade, confirmed by colonialism, exacerbated by fundamental-ism and culminated in an overt civil war which has been raging, with brief interruptions, since 1955.

The ecology of Southern Sudan is such as to make only quite specific ways of life possible. Temperature and rainfall oscillate between extremes and the landscape is extremely flat. The mud dries up and cracks during the dry seasons but is actually flooded during the rainy seasons, so that only the construction of very limited and temporary hamlets on slightly more elevated pieces of land is possible. Except in a few favorable locations, permanent habitation throughout the year is not possible on the plains, which makes migration and pastoral economy a necessity. An almost horizontal portion of the river Nile that creates large swamps, seasonally covered by high grass, traverses the area. These impenetrable areas, the *Sudd*, cut the area off from the outside world until the end of the 19th century. During its very slow flow between its sources in central Africa and its descent in the Cataracts, the White Nile loses more than half of its water by evapora-tion in the extremely hot climate. Canals and dams to regulate the flow (the Jonglei project) are projected in order to make possible the irrigation of large cotton plantations in the Sudan and to increase and control the flow in the Egyptian Nile (Lako 1985). Such measures, however, threaten to exterminate the very basis of the Dinka pastoral culture and form another important reason for the north/south conflict and civil war.

2. THE DINKA

As a people, the Dinka (like the related Nuer) have developed a culture that enables them to survive by an efficient adaptation to the stern restrictions posed by the existing ecological conditions. This adaptation includes a dominantly pastoral economy based primarily on special hump-backed cattle, a migrant way of living and specific structures of social life, ranging from the relations between parent and child and man and woman to the organization of clans and tribes. It also includes a way of socializing children that is both an effect of these conditions and a necessity in order to survive under them. Evans-Pritchard (1940/1994) refers to this as an example of environmental determinism, though of course a literally deterministic model of the relation between culture and personality is today rejected as too simplistic.

For the Dinkas, cattle are not just property but an object of devotion. Apart from their importance for alimentation, they also play a role in the regulation of dowries and the setting-up of families, the social organization and balance of power, and in poetry and other channels of emotional outlet (Deng 1973). If real cattle are not to hand, as for the Dinka living in exile, virtual cattle will be invented to regulate social relations. Money earned in waged labor is considered as different from cattle money. It can be used to pay for everyday commodities but is useless for such matters as dowries and the regulation of social conflicts.

Since time immemorial the Dinka have shaped their culture while driving herds of cattle seasonally between watering and grazing lands. Their lot was to wander over large distances on the plains, exposed to a harsh, unfriendly environment and attacks from wild animals and enemy tribes. It is the boys and young men who tend the cattle. Basically the culture puts two demands on them (Deng 1972): (1) to be stoic and aggressive enough to be able to follow the cattle for lengthy periods and distances under harsh conditions, and to withstand attacks from enemies and wild animals, yet (2) to be controllable by the society, in particular by their fathers.

It seems plausible that the conditions of child rearing among the Dinkas help to create a behavior that can meet these demands. A Dinka boy will spend the first years of his life in his mother's family. His uncle (the mother's brother) becomes his emotional father. These years will stay with him as a memory of closeness and feelings of love, intimacy and fragility. Soon, as early as 4-6 years of age, the boy moves to his father's house and new realities encourage the creation of that shell. He is gradually trained to withstand extreme physical pain through various quite harsh *rites de passage,* ranging from the removal of the mandibular incisive teeth to the painful initial rites marking the passage from adolescence to manhood. The young man is expected to be proud and stoic, capable of endurance and aggressiveness.

Early in life boys begin to tend cattle and as they grow up, they stay a long way away from their parents taking the cattle to the grasslands and protecting them. The girls generally remain closer to home with the women, although girls have roles of great symbolic value (for example in milking the cows). The boys live in the cattle camps accompanied by young men and a few adult traditional leaders. At the beginning of the season they create small groups, but as times goes by these merge into groups of hundreds or thousands of boys and youngsters, their cattle and the traditional leaders. At this time the boys come close to each other: they gather around the fires at night to tell stories, form age sets, unite to care for and defend the cattle, and ultimately develop a culture of warriors prepared to deal with cattle-raiding and attacks by enemies.

This social organization and culture is a way of creating common strength and protection against threats and enemies, a social support which provides food, water, protection and warmth, and a source of courage, emotional security, closeness and friendship. The group behavior and mental structures that are fostered in this way, proves to be very efficient in coping with the stresses of flight and war.

These capable and independent boys are naturally a potential threat to the social hierarchy and to the power of the older men. To maintain the balance there have to be mechanisms of control, and cattle play an important role in these. According to Dinka beliefs, the family has a kind of eternal life thorough procreation. To create a family and to raise children who bear forth the family name is thus a prime goal of life. A person is definitely dead only when no one can recall his name. A man can only pay dowry for a wife by exchange of cattle. The amount of cattle needed is so great that he has to rely on many relatives to provide a share of it. In this way they invest in him, as a result of which he becomes dependent on them -especially on his father. The boy is thus obliged to obey his relatives and his father; he is like a fierce but tamed ox. There is thus a balance between affection and aggressiveness, between the egoistic and the social. Needless to say if there are other ways of arranging a dowry, such as waged labor, or if there are neither cattle nor brides, as in a boys' refugee camp, this balance can become upset (Deng 1972).

The Dinkas have a way of describing the balance between the aggressive and the compassionate, the egoistic and the social - in other words, the world in harmony. When things are in balance the world is in accordance with *cieng*. The accompanying feeling is *adheeng. Cieng* literally means home, a place and a situation where things are well-known, in unity and harmony, as opposed to places and situations where things are not so. It is a concept of ideal human relations. It starts in the relations and good manners in the family but acquires, in the context of the wider society, the meaning of law. As circles widen it becomes blurred, aggressiveness being acceptable against peoples that are foreign to the Dinka. The pride and honour of a human being - related to *cieng* - is called *dheng*. Deng (1972) translates this in terms of nobility, beauty, elegance, charm, graceful- ness, good manners, kindness, singing and dancing. *Dheng* in a way relates to individual- ity and *cieng* to sociability, but only seemingly so - there could not be *dheng* without *cieng,* which brings us back to the balance.

Every young boy gets an ox from his father. The ox represents the boy, his inherent strength that has to be controlled. It is also the representation of the cattle now owned by his father that will once be his own. The boy forces the horns to grow in a delicate and beautiful way. The ox is named after its color pattern. The boy sings poetic songs to his ox. The poems deal with anything from the envy of his father's power, the beauty of girls, the sufferings of hunger and thirst when tending cattle, to the feeling of defeat in love affairs. These songs that exists in many forms, are ways of by-passing the taboo on showing emotions and of complaining and lamenting; they are the direct contact with the emotional self.

2.1. The Unaccompanied Minors

Among the Sudanese refugees pouring into Ethiopia in 1986-87 was a group of around 15,000 boys aged 5-15 years, accompanied by only a few hundred adults. They had fled from armed attacks on their villages or when their families were killed while they were away with the cattle. They also fled from the misery, drought and famine to get shelter and education and the SPLA guerrilla probably sent some away to security in Ethiopia, where they could still remain under considerable control due to the friendly relationship between SPLA and the then Ethiopian regime.

The boys had been trekking for months, sometimes from remote parts of southern Sudan and often with practically no food or water, attacked by wild animals and Arab militia or Sudanese soldiers. They swam over several crocodile-infested rivers. It has been estimated that up to 30% may have succumbed en route. During their travel they formed large groups for support, just as when tending cattle. The groups showed great stability over time.

In Pignudo and Itang in the Gambella region they built their own communities with only limited support from aid organizations. In each hut lived a group of boys that had fled together. The huts were grouped together to form aggregations of 200-300 boys, who were also acquainted since the flight. They built schools and the few adults that had accompanied them served as teachers. It was essentially a refugee community, not a camp build by helpers. Soon various aid organizations provided material support, teach- ing material and medical supplies. The Swedish NGO Radda Barnen set up a mental health team and an interview was carried out with almost all of the minors.

Life went on for five years. When the government of Mengistu in Ethiopia was overthrown and a regime friendly to the Sudanese government took over, the boys had to flee once more. In May 1991 they crossed the flooded river Gilo, were attacked by the Sudanese army and unfriendly tribes, and migrated -mostly on foot- to northern Kenya, which they reached in June 1992 after more than a year en route. They built a new society in Kakuma on the Turkana plains, where they still live the same way, mostly in the same groups that initially fled from the Sudan.

There has been a fierce discussion about the minors being under unwarranted influences. Human Rights Watch (1994) has accused the SPLA of running the camps and using them to recruit soldiers to war against the Sudanese government. The SPLA has certainly had a great influence, especially in Pignudo during the Mengistu era in Ethiopia, and there were undoubtedly some boys who more or less willingly joined the guerrilla. The registration of the boys present in school and during their flight from Ethiopia to Kenya makes it unlikely that large numbers of boys could have been forcibly recruited. One may also consider the possibility that some boys actually are friendly to the cause of the SPLA. Joining the guerrilla is of course an option open to them, even if others consider it to be wrong. The influence of Christian churches and missionaries has been great, a large number of boys converting to Christianity -whether by conviction, for consolation or because of undue influence is hard to say. Finally there is the influence of the helpers' culture. There has been a serious discussion within the camp as to whether the generation growing up are really Dinka or United Nation's High Commission for refugees' (UNHCR) children.

3. EARLIER STUDIES AND CLINICAL EXPERIENCES

At the time of our study certain observations regarding the mental health of the minors had already been made:

1. The Ethiopian teams of Radda Barnen had lived close to the children ever since their arrival in Ethiopia. They had followed them through the Sudan and into the Kakuma camp in Kenya. They had jointly organized emergency support, health care, mental health programs and education.

In 1988-90 this team organized interviews with the children with the double aim of gathering information that could be used for reuniting families and identifying urgent mental health needs. A total of 13,356 of these interviews were carried out by trained interviewers from the Dinka tribe under the supervision of professional Ethiopian psychologists.

Table 1. Symptoms among 1264 children (7-18 years) in the Pignodu camp 1988.

	rarely/never %	sometimes %	always/mostly %
Headache	29	4	3
Recurrent abdominal pains	43	52	4
Fell unhappy	39	58	3
Problems falling asleep	58	39	2
Nightmares	43	55	2
Fearful	63	29	1

Additional structured mental health interviews covering another 27 items were held with 1264 boys in the Pignodu camp (Radda Barnen 1994). These interviews showed that 94% of the children attended school or kindergarten, 94% took part in recreational activities and the majority had helped to build the camp, the living quarters and the schools. 97% stated that they had a best friend, 81% had a good friend among the adults and 82% had somebody to share their troubles with.

The interviews with the sample of 1264 children also asked questions about certain mental and psychosomatic symptoms. As Table 1 shows, it is difficult to draw any firm conclusions about the mental health of the children based on the basis of this study, since most of them fell into the middle category. However, one can safely say that few children appeared to be suffering from severe symptoms.

The clinical experience of the mental health team in the Pignodu camp has also been documented (Radda Barnen 1994). The mental health unit had a hut of their own where treatment and/or counseling could be given to the children when it was deemed necessary. Approximately one percent (173 children, and of these only four more than once) received some form of treatment from the mental health unit. The resources available could have provided treatment for a far greater number. The report also tells of the general impression of the Radda Barnen staff who stayed with the children in Pignudo: that the children were going to school, cooking their food in small groups, playing football, building their houses and schools, and were eager to discuss things.

2. In 1993 a UNICEF team interviewed 174 children in Nasir and Kakuma to evaluate exposure to trauma and its effects (Raundalen et al. 1994). All the children had experienced potentially traumatizing events. 96 children were found to be troubled by traumatic memories and were interviewed more in depth with an adapted version of the 'Impact of events scale' (Horowitz, Wilner, & Alvarez 1979). Eighty-eight percent of the children interviewed were from the original group in Pignodu, 9% had joined the camp during the last 6 months and 3% had just arrived in Kakuma. Intrusive memories as well as avoidant behaviors were very common among the 97 children found to suffer from post-traumatic memories. Of a possible score of 27 on the scale used, the mean score was as high as 21. In a press release, UNICEF declared:

> All the children reported having vivid images of war events. Although the most vivid disturbing after-effects were visual, the most common feature were sounds... They could vividly hear the sounds now. (UNICEF 1993).

Thus at the time when the present study was planned there were two very different views of the state of the children's mental health. The Radda Barnen team stressed the children's ability to cope, whereas the UNICEF team described them as a group in need of extensive intervention because of post-traumatic stress. Radda Barnen decided that a third series of interviews was therefore necessary to shed further light on these conflicting views.

The authors of this article, as independent researchers with an interest in the mental health of refugee children, were assigned to carry out this study on the understanding that they had complete freedom in study design, interpretation of results and scientific publication.

A thorough description of the methods used, including the questionnaire, and the results in full have been presented in a separate report (Jeppsson 1997). In this article we will concentrate on the most important points.

4. THE CURRENT STUDY

4.1. Method

The creation of a questionnaire for the study started with discussions with representatives of the minors, the Sudanese caretakers and the aid personnel. The aim was explained to be to describe the effect of memories of organized violence on the mental health of the children and how the children coped with these memories in a way that would make sense to the boys themselves as well as to Western mental health professionals. In these discussions relevant culture-specific concepts regarding mental health were looked for as well as Western child psychiatric signs and symptoms that made sense in the context of Dinka culture and life in the Kakuma camp. Concepts from a social-construct theory of traumatic stress (McCann & Pearlmann 1990) regarding future perspectives and meaning attributed to traumatic events were introduced, and different ways of finding comfort and support in the camp as well as in traditional Dinka life looked for. On the basis of the information obtained a series of interviews with twenty minors was undertaken with open questions related to these themes. Based on these open interviews a questionnaire was created with a mixture of questions with pre-coded outcomes and open questions. The pre-coded items were constituted of revised open questions where the responses fell in a limited number of easily defined categories. This questionnaire was tested in a small series of pilot interviews and marginally revised again before use in the study population. The complete questionnaire is available from the authors (Jeppsson 1997). The pre-coded questions used very broad categories since it was not possible to use a back-translation technique that would have allowed more subtle categorizations. The open-ended questions were analyzed qualitatively by organizing the responses according to the major themes.

Precoded variables:
- Name, age, origin, name of color bull, occupation at home
- Social network and social support at home and at present, breaks and continuity
- Psychological health, PTSD-related symptoms, their extent and impact on daily life
- *Cieng* and *adheng*

Postcoded variables:
- Self image
- Expectations and wishes for the future
- Meaning ascribed to suffering
- Reasons for leaving, traumatic experiences
- Reasons for unhappiness and feelings of insecurity

Dinka interpreters under the supervision of the investigators carried out the interviews in October-November 1993, in the open air in the camp. The interpreters were generally grown up Dinka men, mostly teachers or administrators employed by Radda Barnen. These men had lived for years with the children, initially fleeing with them in the Sudan.

4.2. Sample

147 children were selected at random from all 26 living quarters, and all of those selected agreed to participate. The mean age was 14 years with an age span of 10 - 18 years. 120 of the 147 children (82%) fell within the range 13-16 years, which prevented an analysis of the importance of age for the different outcomes.

4.3. Results

4.3.1. Background in Sudan

Ninety percent of the children had traditional Dinka backgrounds and only 25% had had any schooling before becoming refugees. 80% had previously tended cattle at home and 83% could name their color bull. 79% had spent time away from their parents in the cattle camps before becoming refugees.

Seventy-six percent named their parents as their main source of comfort in the Sudan; 54% named their father alone. 68% said they missed both parents very much. One third of those interviewed were certain that at least one of their support persons at home was dead, but the majority was unsure of their fates.

4.3.2. Social Network in the Kakuma Camp

Approximately one third of the boys had at least one important support person from home in the camp. The boys still lived in groups of 3-7 per room. The continuity of networks was high and 84% knew at least one of the boys in the hut from Pignudo. With the exception of two, they all said that they were good friends with their cohabitants and 97% spoke of a best friend. 81% said they had good friends among the adults too.

4.3.3. Mental Health

Ninety percent of the children said that their current lifestyle was in accordance with the traditional concepts of cieng and adheng (see above).

4.3.4. Traumatic Events

In the interviews the boys talked about the extreme hardships they had experienced; the death of loved ones, war scenes of killings, rapes and mutilations; attacks by wild animals; people drowning, hunger and disease. Some of these events had taken place in the home village, but many also during their walks to and from the two campsites (Table 2).

Table 2. Terrible events mentioned by the children in the interviews

Death
- death of father and mother
- death of brother
- death of relatives at home
- killing of uncles
- suicide
- drowning of some of the children in the river

War scenes
- shot by Anuak at Pochalla
- massacre of children by Anuak of Ethiopia
- the massacre of some of the children by Toposas
- gun fights
- gun battles
- attempt to kill
- rape
- the dreadful Gilo war
- air raids

Wild animals
- friends eaten by lions
- children killed in attacks by wild animals

Hunger and disease
- hunger on the way to Pignudo
- dying of thirst
- being sick on the way to Kacoma

4.3.5. Symptoms related to post-traumatic suffering

Intrusive memories To get an idea of the extent to which the children were troubled by their memories they were asked if they often or seldom had nightmares or were bothered by these thoughts during the day. 20% of the children reported that they often had nightmares and/or difficulties getting to sleep when they had nightmares. 16% were frequently bothered by their thoughts during the day, while only 5% of the whole group reported that they were so preoccupied that it prevented them from playing or doing school work.

Eighty percent of the children gave examples of how they coped with troubling memories. 34% of the boys described different religious practices; such as going to church and talk to the priest, reading the bible or praying. Another 30% described seeking comfort from either a friend in the camp or a trusted adult. Less common examples were playing or reading a book (10%) or going to school (7%).

Mood   Only 2% of the children reported feeling sad most of the time. 90% reported that they sometimes felt happy and sometimes sad, while 5% stated that they were happy most of the time.

When asked what caused them to feel sad, 30% mentioned memories. The other 70% attributed their sadness to other causes such as being away from home or longing for their family (22%), the war itself or news related to the war (18%) or problems in the camp such as fights between the boys (14%).

When asked to whom they could go to when they felt sad, 91% named someone, in most cases a friend (35%), a caretaker (24%) or a relative (20%).

When asked about what or whom in the camp that made them feel happy the majority mentioned school or education (62% of all) as a source of happiness, followed by playing (18%) and being together with others in the group (10%).

Fears   Thirty-three percent admitted being afraid at times. The fear most often mentioned was for attacks in the camp, followed by a fear of loud sounds and wild animals. The more unspecific fear of darkness was rarely mentioned.

Meaning   The boys were asked if they thought there was any meaning or reason behind the violent events they had experienced, and if so what reason this might be. Only 9% said they felt the war had a definite meaning. 36% gave a straight no and the remaining majority said they were not sure. 37% felt that they had been unlucky, which might also reflect a sense of the war having no meaning.

The two dominant themes of explanation in the interviews were religion and the struggle for freedom. 44% interpreted the war and related events within a political framework. A few of these children did express a strong political commitment, but greater number gave vague answers like they say it is for freedom.

The Christian faith seemed to have a strong influence on the world-view of the boys. 96% stated that they believed in God and 90% expressed the belief that God could help them. Almost 30% of the boys gave explanations to the war that within this religious framework, where the war was interpreted as an act of God, either as a punishment or with a divine meaning beyond the realm of humans.

Self-image   All the children said they knew at least one thing they were good at, in most cases schoolwork or sports. 85% expressed confidence in their schoolwork by saying that they felt most school assignments were easy. 98% said they felt they were a good person to be with. Only 3% reported feeling inferior to the others.

Perspective on the future   The children's outlook on the future was quite positive. Fifteen years from now they expected to have formed a family (96%), to have children (93%), to have a job (96%) and have cattle (90%). However, there seemed to be a lot of uncertainty regarding their own long-term survival, since as many as 62% were doubtful if they would be alive fifteen years on.

The majority believed they would live in peace as adults, but as many as 31% expressed doubts about this. There was a great deal of uncertainty among the boys as to whether they would be reunited with their families: only 10% were certain they would see their family again, 72% were uncertain, and 12% said they were certain that they would never see their family again.

When asked about future job plans, many said they hoped to become skilled professionals such as doctors (17%), teachers (16%), priests (7%) or engineers (4%) through university studies. Many expressed an intention to combine this career with a traditional Dinka life, while only 13% said they expected to lead a wholly traditional Dinka life. Only one child mentioned the ambition to become a soldier.

Wishes for the Future Lastly, the boys were asked about their wishes for the future. A fair number hoped to become skilled professionals, while many expressed a longing to be back with their parents and family in the Sudan. The majority expressed altruistic hopes, like peace in the Sudan or even the world, and the desire to help their fellow men. No one expressed a desire for revenge.

5. DISCUSSION

The results of the above study seem to stress the importance of going beyond a narrow trauma discourse in mental health programs for refugee children in a non-Western context. A UNICEF team demonstrated a high incidence of traumatic events and PTSD among the Sudanese boys who were refugees in Kakuma (Raundalen et al., 1994). Our own results confirmed that these symptoms were widespread, but seemed to indicate a surprisingly limited impact on the boys' daily life and well-being. Another aspect of the PTSD concept within this context, which is highlighted here, is the adaptive nature of hypervigilance and fears in a dangerous environment. For these children, brought up to protect their cows from wild animals and hostile neighbors, it seems rather doubtful whether hypervigilance should be considered a pathological symptom requiring treatment. There were also few signs of the developmental consequences which would be expected within a Western theoretical framework from exposure to such a violent environment (Garbarino, 1991). Future outlooks were fairly bright given the harsh living conditions, and few children reported having problems at school. The finding that many children doubted if they would be alive 15 years from now could be interpreted as a sign of a depressive worldview. However, within the context of life in southern Sudan during the last decades, it is also quite possible that this should rather be interpreted as a rational estimate of the possibilities of long-term survival in this region.

Every definition of mental health is bound to a given cultural context. A classic definition in Western psychology is that given by Sigmund Freud: a sane person is one who is capable of love and work. In Kakuma 98% of the children felt that somebody liked them. Their dreams for the future consisted of building a better life for their country and mankind; the desire for revenge or to become a soldier was not expressed. There was a sense of self-reliance and a feeling of friendship and acceptance among comrades. There was a feeling of trust in human beings and an ability to confide in friends and adults. As a whole, the children seemed to possess a great ability for love. And they had worked hard: with the help of their caretakers, they themselves had built the camp in which they lived in Pignodu; they harvested their own crops, fished in the river and walked for many miles. Above all, they had been attending school and enjoying it. In a Dinka context, a more appropriate definition of mental health would be based on whether life was in accordance with *cieng* and *adheng*. According to 90% of the children it was. Finally we have the impression of the Radda Barnen mental health team who worked in the camp for many years and who failed to find the mental disturbances they were employed to treat.

How can we understand the ability of these boys to cope with the extremely stressful events they had experienced? One may speculate that evolution has promoted a particular form of socialization as an efficient means of surviving the harsh conditions of life in southern Sudan. We have discussed above how this socialization tends to promote a certain type of mental structure and group behavior, which are favourable in a life of following and defending animals in a harsh environment. This certainly also made it possible for the boys to survive many months of movement through the very hostile war zones in southern Sudan. Beneath the tough exterior Dinka culture provides emotional outlets that are valuable in dealing with difficult experiences in life. Poetry, empathy, close friendship and a sense of solidarity within the group all provide access to this emotional self and an ability to share and deal with the difficult experiences. The group behavior of the young Dinkas certainly forms a double-edged defense against both wild animals and attacking rival tribes. The mutual emotional support mechanisms within the group are a prerequisite to surviving and relating in a healthy way to the harsh realities in the plains of southern Sudan, as well as to the extremely tragic events the boys lived through during the civil war and their flight.

If the culture-specific group behavior of the Dinka minors is as important as we are suggesting, one must praise the organization of the camp for creating a culture-sensitive structure. Partly due to a lack of resources in the barren Ethiopian countryside and partly due to the wisdom of the aid personnel, these structures and way of life were left alone. The boys were allowed to remain in their groups. Attempts to intervene, to break down the groups and place individual boys with foster families, were thwarted. The boys were also left in charge of building and organizing their society, houses, schools, and activities. This meant they remained the subjects of their lives and did not become objects, passively assisted refugees. This has probably been a key factor in protecting these boys from the social construction of victimization (Swartz & Levett, 1989). Wolf & Fesseha (1998) have described the importance of a democratic and supportive environment for the mental health of orphans in institutions in Eritrea. These findings suggest that a camp structure like that in Kakuma or Pignodu is beneficial to the mental health of orphaned refugee children regardless of cultural context.

The present study also demonstrates the shortcomings of a simplified anthropological approach to studies of refugee children under the strong influence of Western NGOs. No more than 25% of the boys had been to school at all before becoming refugees, and now 44% of the boys envisioned a future that involved a university education. These boys, who had been raised to herd cattle in an animistic culture, now express strong Christian beliefs. As one Dinka representative put it: "These boys don't belong to the Dinkas any more, their culture is UNICEF".

Punamaeki (1996) described the importance of a strong political/nationalist conviction for Israeli children to be able to cope with political violence. However, there was no obvious indication in the present study that a political framework was very important for the Dinka boys. Most boys gave vague answers that could be interpreted as a way of dissociating themselves from the political struggle. It is also quite possible that these vague answers were the boys' way of shrugging off a difficult question. However, it seems that Christian religious ideas were more important for the boys in their construction of a meaning. Before entering the camp in Pignodu, the majority of the boys had animist beliefs; now they believed in a Christian God and quite a few even mentioned becoming a priest as a serious job option. This transformation must be explained in light of the strong presence of Christian missionaries in the Kakuma camp, but may also have a political significance in relation to the Moslem enemy in the Sudan conflict.

This study has some obvious methodological shortcomings. The limited funding available and the expectations of Radda Barnen to have fairly quick results for use in their work with the boys prevented us from using interview and observation techniques that would have allowed us to gain a more profound understanding of the world view and belief systems of the boys and how these related to the boys' coping with their memories of organized violence. The lack of a back-translation check means that some inaccuracies in the translation may have affected the results (Brislin, 1983). There was also a risk involved in using camp interpreters as interviewers, since responses could have been biased by a fear that they might be used against the children later on. It is also possible that the interpreters themselves may have biased the information by withholding some of the material given to them by the children, since the interviews can be seen as an evaluation of the work which they have participated in for several years.

The particular political situation of the camp should be taken into account when considering the boys' thoughts about their future and the meaning of the war. For an outside observer it is very difficult to estimate the amount of political pressure the boys were subjected to. It is quite possible that the fact that so few aspired to becoming soldiers is a reflection of the fear that such answers could be useful for the enemies of the SPLA. But if the camp were under guerrilla influence, as some have suggested, it is quite remarkable that so many boys expressed doubts about the meaning of the war. It is hard to imagine that these responses would be of any use to the SPLA. The only certain conclusion that can be drawn is that research in this context is easily influenced by the political realities at hand. The investigators were clearly related to Radda Barnen, which had followed and supported the boys for years and was thus trusted. On the other hand the organization was of course close to the camp management and this implied substantial control over the boys' future. Since it is impossible to measure the effects of any of the above circumstances, the results should be interpreted carefully.

Maybe it is easier to become aware of the importance of the cultural context in the present setting because the Dinka culture is so exotic and the events of the south Sudanese conflict so extreme. In another recent study, Englund (1998) described how Mozambican refugees in Malawi use traditional rituals to cope with war trauma. Cultural context is probably just as important under less exotic and therefore less obvious circumstances. These two studies therefore seem to add another dimension to the controversy regarding the content of psycho-social programs in refugee work (Richman, 1993; Kuterovac & Dyregrov, 1994; Boyden, 1994; Bracken, 1995; Stubbs & Soroya, 1996; Editorial, 1997; Summerfield 1999). Western psychology and psychiatry are not the only remedies for the suffering of victims of war and political repression. It is therefore important that mental health workers in refugee work have a thorough knowledge of the cultural context in which they are performing. Otherwise they run the risk not only of limiting their repertoire of ways of offering support, but of actually replacing existing coping skills with ones which are less effective in that particular context.

REFERENCES

Boyden, J. (1994) Children's experience of conflict related emergencies: some implications for relief policy and practice. *Disasters 18*, 254-267.

Bracken, P., Giller, J., & Summerfield, D. (1995) Psychological responses to war and atrocity: the limitations of current concepts. *Social Science & Medicine 40*, 1073-1082.

Brislin, R. (1983) Cross-cultural research in psychology. *Annual Review of Psychology 34*, 363-400.

Deng, F. (1973) *Dinka and their Songs*. Oxford: Clarendon.

Deng, F. M (1972) *The Dinka of the Sudan*. New York: Holt, Rinehart and Winston.

Editorial (1997) The uses of psychosocial epidemiology in promoting refugee health. *American Journal of Public Health 87*, 726-728.

Englund, H. (1998) Death, trauma and ritual Mozambican refugees in Malawi. *Social Science & Medicine 46*, 1165-1174.

Evans-Pritchard, E. (1940/1994) *The Nuer*. London: Clarendon Press.

Garbarino, J. (1991) Developmental consequences of living in dangerous and unstable environments: the situation of refugee children. In: M. McCallin (ed.), *The psychological well-being of refugee children. Research practice and policy issues*. Geneva: International Catholic Child Bureau, 2-18.

Horowitz, M., Wilner, N., & Alvarez, W. (1979) Impact of Event Scale: a measure of subjective stress. *Psychosomatic Medicine 41*, 209-218.

Human Rights Watch (1994) *Civilian Devastation. Abuses by all Parties in the War in Southern Sudan*. New York, Human Rights Watch/Africa.

Jeppsson, O. (1997) *Traumatic Stress in Cultural Context - a Study of Unaccompanied Refugee Children from Southern Sudan*. Stockholm: Child and Adolescent Public Health Unit.

Kuterovac, G., & Dyregrov, A. (1994) A silent majority under stress. *British Journal of Medical Psychology 67*, 375-379.

Lako, G. (1985) The impact of the Jonglei scheme on the economy of the Dinka *African Affairs 84*, 15-38.

McCann, I. L., & Pearlmann, L. A. (1990) *Psychological Trauma and the Adult Survivor. Theory, Therapy and Transformation*. New York: Brunner/Mazel.

Punamaeki, R. (1996) Can ideological commitment protect children's psychological well-being in situations of political violence? *Child Development 67*, 55-69.

Radda Barnen (1994) *The Unaccompanied Minors of Southern Sudan*. Skara: Radda Barnen.

Raundalen, M., Dyregrov, A., Derib, A., Juma, F., & Kassa, S. (1994) *A Treatment Study of the Unaccompanied Minors from the Southern Sudan*. Nairobi: UNICEF.

Summerfield, D. (1999) A critique of seven assumptions behind psychological trauma programmes in war affected areas. *Social Science & Medicine 48*, 1449-1462.

Stubbs, P., & Soroya, B. (1996) War trauma, psychosocial projects and social development in Croatia. *Medicine, Conflict & Survival 12*, 303-14.

Swartz, L., & Levett, A. (1989) Political repression and children in South Africa: The social construction of damaging effects. *Social Science & Medicine 287*, 741-750.

UNICEF (1993) *Addressing the Needs of War-traumatized Children in South-Sudan*. Nairobi: UN Operation Life Line Sudan, Southern sector.

Wolf, P., & Fesseha, G. (1998) The orphans of Eritrea: Are orphanages part of the problem or part of the solution? *American Journal of Psychiatry 155*, 1319-1324.

5. MEETING THE MENTAL HEALTH NEEDS OF CHILDREN WHO HAVE BEEN ASSOCIATED WITH FIGHTING FORCES
Some lessons from Sierra Leone

Ian Clifton-Everest[1]

Ibrahim is 12 years old. He was abducted in the east of Freetown in January 1999 at the time of the incursion of the RUF.[2] According to him, he is from the North of Sierra Leone, but at that time he was staying in a displaced persons' camp with his parents, who were murdered at the time of his abduction. Ibrahim was discharged from the military three weeks ago and is now in the 'interim care center' managed by COOPI.[3] There, he spends long periods in solitude, separated from his friends. He seems very anxious and unwell. He complains that he was drugged by his captors and that he now suffers severe after-effects. He has terrible headaches which he attributes to the drugs administered to him through an incision in his temple, and to the imminent justice awaiting him for the bad things he was forced to do by his captors. Sometimes afraid, he talks mystically about things that he saw or sees; rather as though he was having hallucinations.

1. CHILDREN AND WAR IN SIERRA LEONE

The civil conflict in Sierra Leone lasted twelve years. Like many other wars in Africa, it was a complex one. For much of the time it was low-keyed, but its intensity fluctuated, as uneasy periods of peace gave way to new rounds of fighting, as new power groups emerged to replace old ones, and as existing factions realigned into new alliances. The war has left little room for a clear division between soldier and civilian, child and adult. Much of the population has found itself at some time or another bound in service to fighting factions, including many children, some lured with promises of reward, others drawn in because they no longer had family to support them, and yet others forcibly abducted by fighting factions as a mark of their domination over town and village.

---

[1] Ian Clifton-Everest, Senior Lecturer, London Metropolitan University.
[2] Revolutionary United Front.
[3] Italian non-governmental organization, *Cooperazione Internazionale*.

It can be said with some confidence that more than 10,000 children served under the command of fighting forces in Sierra Leone. The exact figure will never be known, since many children never underwent any formal process of demobilization, and families would be unlikely to give honest information about the involvement of their children at any census. Based simply on numbers of children reported by their families as missing in 2001, it was estimated that some 5,400 children still remain mobilized with fighting forces. The figure was at the very best approximate, since there was no obvious way to make the necessary correction for the number of families that did not – or could not – report that their children were missing. Nor was it possible to estimate the proportion of missing children who were dead or living with other relatives, rather than in active service. Nevertheless, if to this figure is added the 2,500 children that were released from service with fighting forces during the previous 18 months, and the many more children released in earlier cycles of demobilization, it becomes clear that many thousands of children must have experienced life in the service of armed factions in Sierra Leone. What have been the experiences of these children, and how have their experiences impacted on them in their formative years? What are the mental health issues raised by these experiences and what kinds of psychosocial programs are needed to address them?

2. IDENTIFYING THE RIGHT FORMS OF MENTAL HEALTH INTERVENTION

Policies for demobilizing children associated with fighting forces in Sierra Leone placed considerable stress on the mental health care of recently released children. Guidelines established jointly by the Ministry of Social Welfare, UNAMSIL and UNICEF emphasized the need for careful monitoring of mental health both prior to and after reunification with the families. Support programs were also required to help children come to terms with experiences of the past and readjust to civilian and family life. Many of the children released by fighting factions following the Lome Peace Accord in 1999 were reunified with family in the Freetown area where much of the country's population were sheltering in displaced persons' camps. Upon their release most children were cared for in reception centers run by the Italian NGO *Cooperazione Internazionale* (COOPI) and the local NGO Family Homes Movement. These agencies documented the children, traced their families, and arranged for their reunification. The same NGO's were also responsible for following the children up after they had been reunified with their families – or in some cases, after they were placed in alternative care. Drawing on information obtained by these agencies through the use of questionnaires, behavioral rating scales, structured interviews and observational schedules, it is possible to obtain some useful insights into the mental health needs of these children.

Mental health professionals are inclined to approach the problems of children who have been caught up in war with concepts like trauma, stress and distress. Most usually they work with the assumption that such children have been through events that they have found highly frightening and difficult to comprehend. Persisting memories of the events continue to distress them for some time afterwards, and may disrupt behavior, thought and capacity to live a normal life. Among the behaviors that are often associated with such reactions to trauma, are episodes of weeping, isolation, sleep disorders, nightmares, enuresis.

Certainly, among children in interim care centers and among those returned to their families in Freetown, there were some who showed such behaviors; but the frequency of these stress signs may not be that much greater than would be found in any group of children entering a new and unfamiliar institution such as a reception center. The issue of whether children do show intense and lasting distress in response to experiences they have undergone while serving with armed factions is an important one, and one we shall come back to. For the moment, let it be said that – in the eyes of those who care for the children from day to day – it is not behaviors normally considered indices of trauma and stress that are the most troubling, nor the ones in need of the most urgent attention. Much more striking is:

- Uninhibitedly aggressive and threatening behavior that is used to gain the upper hand, and extract from the staff whatever is wanted.
- Deep distrust of adults, and derisive contempt of most offers of help.
- Pronounced worries about personal security and the possibility of betrayal to those who might take revenge for atrocities committed in the past.
- Refusal to return to their communities for fear that their families will be unwilling to, or to accept the fact that there villages have been destroyed.
- Deep confusion about the rights and wrongs of past actions – with some show of remorse, but more frequent boasting of atrocities committed.
- A conviction that thieving is the only possible way of getting what you need in life.

Do these behaviors raise mental health issues? Certainly we do not have to assume the children are suffering from mental illness to explain them. In many ways, their behaviors and feelings are highly rational. They have served the children well for life in the bush, and with the continuing insecurity in the country may well give them equally good protection in the foreseeable future. For these reasons, we certainly cannot call their behaviors maladjusted. Much as those who care for the children would like to see different behaviors that were more trusting, showed greater respect for other people's rights, and were less aggressive, the children cannot be denied the right to behave in ways that ensure their survival in the social context in which they find themselves. The following case-study of a 15-year old boy illustrates the survival strategies a child soldier learns during his career and how those strategies are hampering his reintegration into civil life.

Mohammed was abducted by the RUF at the age of ten and spent three years working for this group before he escaped, to be captured and enrolled again - this time by the SLA.[4] He was demobilized four weeks ago and is now in the 'interim care center' managed by COOPI near Freetown. For Mohammed, his family life memories are far back in the past compared to the memories of the military life he lived for the last five years. His memories of this period are however quite positive. Of course the memories of being separated from his family sometimes cause him sadness, but the hardships of military life did not prevent him from developing good contacts with his superiors and strong friendships with his

---

[4] Sierra Leone Army

comrades. The daily routine of the military gave him a sense of security and in general, he felt well taken care of by his superiors.

Mohammed was not very bothered by his duty to kill the enemy. In his family home, it was customary to hunt predatory animals. His superiors have taught him that to slay the enemy was not different. It is not men that one kills, but sub-humans. When someone thought they had killed an enemy, he would proudly brag about it with his friends. They would listen with admiration and the superiors would celebrate the event. There was no suggestion that anything bad been done. However, Mohammed's life as a combatant has not been without anxiety. We are not talking here about typical childhood anxieties, like family disputes, the threat of famine, diseases, or the 'poro' rituals. We refer to the unpredictability of the violence surrounding him; the imminence of death in an attack (by ECOMOG[5], or the Kamajors, or even the RUF); the contradictory behavior of his superiors who, under the influence of drugs, could become reckless during the attacks, and would commit atrocities not only against the enemy, but also against their own members, and especially against the women. Threats like these often challenged his sense of security and gave him a kind of distrust for everyone around him, especially of adults. Sometimes Mohammed also had anxieties about his future. If the war should end, what would become of him? Should he then return to his family? How would he find his family, as they were surely displaced? Once out of military protection, would he not be at constant risk for retaliations? And how to earn a livelihood in civil life when one has almost no schooling or vocational training?

During his first four weeks in civilian life, his problems have taken bigger and bigger proportions for him, and are now becoming a real obsession. At the time of the demobilization, he did not really think about the future. Facing the need to ensure his own security in a new situation of uncertainties, and without arms, he became completely engrossed in a survival strategy, observing distrustfully all the events happening around him, looking out for any attacks, hiding his identity and avoiding answering any questions that would compromise him. Now, feeling more secure and at ease at the interim care center, he has time to think. COOPI wants to reunify him with his family. Should he cooperate and give the necessary information about his identity? Or should he continue to stall the process and prolong his stay at the center, where his personal security is better ensured? The fact that he does not know where his family is, and the unstable security conditions in different parts of the country, makes this decision even more difficult to take. COOPI talks about dialogue with his family to make them aware of his problems and to help his reintegration. Can he trust this? One thing that he is sure about is that he would like to return to school in order to catch up on the years he lost. Already these last three weeks, he goes to school in the morning and really enjoys it. COOPI, however, insists on reintegrating him in his family before enrolling him in a real school. But when a person returns to his family, should he not do so with pride? Should he not return as a war hero loaded with trophies,

---

[5] Military operation dispatched by the ECOWAS in order to restore peace and stability in Sierra Leone

rather than as a lost son? How to come back without nice fashionable shoes, without any diamonds or reward money? All these things were promised by his superiors at the time of the demobilization, but refused by COOPI since he came to the center.

Other anxieties have also started to trouble Mohammed these last three weeks. How to reconcile the past with the present? The life that stands before him now, and the life he led for the last five years, are like two worlds which do not connect and present contradictions of truth and morality. Three weeks ago, people applauded his participation in atrocities as a moral act. Now he feels that those same actions are regarded as monstrous and pathological. And if they are indeed monstrous and pathological, how can he be held responsible? Where are the limits of his responsibility? Were they actions of free will? Can one be responsible for actions committed in ignorance? Mohammed finds it impossible to confront the future under the load of guilt that is piled up on him and he finds it easier to take refuge in his own morality. With his friends he talks with nostalgia about his life as a combatant as if it was the golden age, and together they try to reconstruct the old military order inside the center as a symbol of distrust against those who want to impose on them new things. It is as if the old morality is made more valid by its simple application within the group.

Back in the solitude of his personal thoughts, Mohammed admits it is not easy to escape such a moral dilemma. All the more so since his superiors are now admitting that they committed atrocities and the top commanders are calling for a spirit of forgiveness. At his demobilization, he felt betrayed by his superiors, who gave up the fight and abandoned him to UNAMSIL. Now he finds himself in the hands of an international NGO whose unfamiliar principle's of humanitarianism and apolitical stance are so different from what he knows and create new uncertainties At the beginning, he controlled his feelings out of concern for retaliation. Over recent days, however, he has felt more and more frustrated and enraged by the betrayal, and a growing sense of security allows him to show it. His violence is not only directed towards his former superiors, but also towards anybody who draws attention to his current dilemma, including those who take care of him at the center. Even worse, his aggressive impulses threatens to engulf his friends and himself. It frightens him.

3. HELPING CHILDREN GLIMPSE A BETTER FUTURE

Creating a new social order in Sierra Leone, an order where children will feel secure to return to their families; where they will see some dividend from a respect for human rights, from treating people courteously, for working for what they want rather than stealing it, is not in the gift of the mental health worker. It requires a political settlement, backed up by a determined effort to establish law and order and other essential institutions of civil society. Arguably, however, there is also a psychological element to any process of social reconstruction, because where the anger, bitterness and sense of loss goes so deep as it does in Sierra Leone, no new order can be achieved without some adjustment of people's mental world. For many, and in particularly for children who were conscripted to serve with the fighting forces, it will require a supreme effort to overcome deep seated feeling of anger, hatred and mistrust that sustain continuing cycles of revenge. It is here that the mental health worker has an important role.

In the political environment of Sierra Leone where the prospects of improved security, and enforcement of law and order still seem far from certain, such a healing process has to be approached with caution, and in full cognizance of continuing social problems. Any support activities that ignores the deep seated injustices and corruption that still pervade every day life are likely to be counter-productive. In most cases they will carry little credibility with children, and when they do, will work against children's interests. It is not a service to develop in these children a misplaced sense of trust in others; an expectation that constructive work will always be fairly rewarded; and that courtesy in human relationships always pays higher dividends than intimidation. But as a matter of human rights, it is never too early for these children to have the opportunity to glimpse the possibility of a more humane world than the one in which they are currently trapped, so they can be freed from the legacy of a psychological trauma which will prevent them from playing a full part in its construction when the time comes.

4. THE COOPI PROGRAM

An example of a program which set out to do just this is the one that COOPI used in its work with recently demobilized children in Freetown during 2001 and 2002. It served as a prelude to a much fuller involvement of children in the promotion of a new order of human rights as the peace became consolidated. The program combined elements of humanistic therapy with peace education and civics. It covered a range of topics concerned with the construction of a better society (e.g. alternatives to stealing; controlling conflict and aggression; managing other people's vindictiveness; helping to rebuild villages etc.). Working in small groups, children used drama, story telling, drawing, music or simple discussion to explore the topics. They were encouraged first to express their fears and anxieties about things as they are, and the changes they would like to see. The sessions then moved on to explore the possible roles of individuals and institutions in bringing about change. Finally children were encouraged through self-reflection to identify beliefs feelings and attitudes, and behaviors of their own that act as barriers to change. To ensure that the program played some role in building real hope for the future, considerable emphasis was placed in each session on the search for a few practical solutions to problems that were of high importance to the children. Children may contribute their own suggestions to questions such as how a foster child should make himself more wanted by foster parents, or what to do if parents start complaining that a child has been away for so long and brought nothing back to the family.

Mohammed has stayed at the COOPI interim care center for four weeks. It may seem contradictory that, coming to a point where he has enough trust to confront the reality of his situation, Mohammed's behavior is now even more difficult than three weeks ago. But already he has made important steps. At the beginning of his stay at the COOPI center, Mohammed maintained a strong distrust towards everybody, a habit gained during his long career as a young combatant. Thanks to the patience and the devotion of those who take care of him at the center, he has gained a renewed trust in human relations, in the capacity of people to unconditionally care for him without putting their own interests before his. Of course, he has at times anxieties about his security, especially when we talk about reunifying him with his family and when we question him about his identity and origin. However, in the center he feels secure. It is the prospect of being set outside, without this new sense of security, that causes him to panic.

The new security order is also an important factor enabling Mohammed to confront the puzzling contradictions of his life. In the beginning he avoided this confrontation, fearing that his disruptive behavior would come back in the form of violent repercussions. Now he has faith that the reasons for his disruptive behavior are understood by those who take care of him, and he feels supported by adults in his attempts to confront problems. If bad behavior is not approved, at least it is tolerated, as long as it does not lead him to violence. Those who are managing the center took care to create a world around him where the limits to what is acceptable and what is not are very well defined. The consequences of bad behavior are thus very predictable. Any behavior that threatens the security of others is strictly forbidden and automatically leads to isolation from others. This definition of the limits and consequences of behavior is a relief for Mohammed. It provides him with a protective structure in which he can explore his personal problems. He knows how far he can go without the risk of his behavior backfiring.

Mohammed is supported in his battle against the contradictions of his life by the caregivers who look after him during the day and by a 'psychosocial worker'. The latter organizes a few individual counseling sessions for him, in which he can express his worries about the future and his conflicting feelings about his past behavior. Just being listened to is important to Mohammed. The psychosocial worker is especially respectful of Mohammed's own perspective and views, and does not try to diminish the importance of his problems. At the same time, the psychosocial worker tries to give a broader perspective on the contradictions, stressing that responsibility is never completely individual, and that if he tries to share Mohammed's anxieties, it is because he also is willing to take some responsibility. He insists on the good things realized by his young client in the past and on the importance of seeing the good and bad as different aspects of his personality. In this way he tries to prevent his client from going into complete self-devaluation and even more destruction. He also tries to prevent Mohammed from denying the actions that trouble him, or from reversing mo-rality, where the bad is again seen as the good... These solutions would be too easy!

Mohammed engages with his friends in group discussions organized by his caregiver. They talk about what they have done, their experiences, their reactions, their feelings and the emotions everybody had. Mohammed is surprised that some of his peers have had the same moments of fear as himself, and were affected by the same experiences. They also talk about the morality of the things they did, and their feelings of guilt. It is also a relief for Mohammed to know that some friends are very troubled by the same thoughts and the same feelings regarding what they have done. It gives him the reassurance that he has the reactions of a normal boy and that he is not going crazy. The group discussion on these issues also reinforces his sense of shared responsibility. If in the future one can share the weight of what one has done, it will seem less heavy. The objective of these therapeutic sessions is always to prepare the youngsters for the future. In so far as there is talk about the past, it is because one cannot be effective in the future while carrying the traumas from the past. In the management of the sessions, the caregivers are closely alert to the danger of children relapsing into nostalgia, confabulation and idealistic reconstructions of the past, which can so easily serve as tactics for avoiding troubling moral issues.

The road towards reunification will be very long for Mohammed, and the goal will be very difficult to reach. As long as he has not enough trust to provide accurate information about his origins, the first steps to trace his family cannot be taken. We try to convince him that he will only be reunified if his security is guaranteed, but he maintains his resistance. Maybe he knows less than we think about his family and their whereabouts. Maybe he is responsible for atrocities within his own family and he does not want to talk about it. Such things are frequently the case. Mohammed will always carry his portion of responsibility for the atrocities committed and this will continue to upset him. But if he can find a role in society in which he can do good things, the past will acquire a less troubling character. A lot will depend on the way he is accepted by the community. The community can either continue to distrust him, or can try to look for reconciliation, maybe even using traditional cleansing rituals to give him absolution. At least Mohammed has started on the road to reintegration in civil life and reconciliation with himself. He will continue to receive the support of the center in his efforts to attain these ends, as long as he needs it.

The program, which was originally piloted with children in interim care, was subsequently adapted for use in schools. Here there was the additional challenge of establishing a dialogue between those who have been conscripted into armed factions, and those who have been victims. To avoid sessions that could be too explosive, it was found necessary to find ways of approaching some of the issues more obliquely rather than head-on. Nevertheless, it proved possible to get children to reflect on feelings and experiences of aggression distrust, vindictiveness, destruction and dishonesty without the risk of embarrassment or threat to individuals or groups who are known to have been involved in atrocities. Schools are an excellent point of departure for achieving impact on the broader community because parents in Freetown take a keen interest in what their children are doing at school. In one school a small group of children developed a piece of drama around the theme of personal responsibility and loyalty to the group. This vividly depicted the dilemma of a child who faced vindictiveness if she broke ranks with her peers and refused to take part in punishing another child who had been identified as a collaborator in some former atrocity. It drew attention to the lack of civil institutions to afford her protection. The small piece so impressed the head-teacher that he had it performed at an assembly in front of the whole school, and as many parents attended as children!

5. HOW IMPORTANT IS PTSD AMONG DEMOBILISED CHILDREN IN SIERRA LEONE?

What challenges can mental health professionals expect to find as they set about this work with children? Down what path does the child have to be taken to get beyond the feelings, beliefs and attitudes that currently trap him? Can he reach the end of the path simply by reasoned instruction, or have events of the past set up some kind of emotional vortex in which the child is swept along, so that he is no longer open to reason – perhaps incapable even of a sustained relationship with those who seek to help him? And will the mental health worker discover other needs that need answering on the way? These questions bring us back to the topic of trauma. For example in the case of Ibrahim.

Ibrahim cannot describe the bad things he did. Maybe he does not remember them very well. Maybe he is too afraid to reconstruct them in his own thoughts. Maybe he is hiding them out of fear of retaliation. Maybe they are imaginary things, things that he was made to believe he had done, so as to make him afraid of retaliation or prevent him from escaping. This kind of blackmail is often used with children. In the past week, Ibrahim has been showing other kinds of disturbed behavior. At times he becomes very agitated, moving from one place to the other, as if he is trying to escape some bothersome thoughts. In this state of agitation, he cannot concentrate on tasks. When we ask him to do something, he gladly begins, but very soon becomes distracted. So it seems that he spends hours doing useless things. He participates in school classes, but as soon as the teacher stops giving him individual attention, he gets no work done. He complains about not having being able to get to sleep, and having stayed awake for long periods at night. We can see that he is sleepy in the morning, but soon he becomes agitated and hyperactive. He is now constantly in the care of the doctor in charge of the children of the center. He already receives two Valium pills in the evening and one in the morning. We hesitate to raise the dosage without going more deeply into his problems. The doctor and the psychosocial worker are working together on it. Referring to the things that he claims to see and to his disturbed behavior, the question we asked ourselves is whether this young boy might have some psychotic disorder. But considering his age and the other circumstances, we were inclined to a different hypothesis. It seems more probable that he had some very bad experiences under the influence of drugs and that he is at times experiencing flashbacks. The restlessness he started to show a few days ago might be caused by some other drugs he obtains from a dealer recently arrived in the village[6].

However, there are still things that we cannot explain very well. Why does Ibrahim get agitated in the morning, while it is in the afternoon that he goes out

---

[6] Children in Sierra Leone have easy access to drugs; many of these are newly imported from neighbouring countries. It is believed that among theses are some natural products until now still unknown in Europe or in The United States. Other drugs are pharmaceutical products, often illegal and of bad quality. The origin of these substances and their nature are however often unknown, even by the local population, and their effects not studied. Thus the behavior of young combatants directly resulting from the use of drugs remains unknown.

into the village? Even more difficult to explain is why Ibrahim would take
stimulants when he is already so anxious.

Children who have experienced atrocities of war are sometimes described as
suffering posttraumatic stress disorder or PTSD (see e.g. Yule & Williams, 1990).
Characteristically, such sufferers continue to be troubled by intrusive thoughts, vivid
flashbacks, or nightmares related to disturbing past events. In some cases the unwanted
intrusions are accompanied by panic attacks. They are often induced by a smell, sight,
and sound or thought that was associated with the past incident. Sufferers may also
continue to be troubled by feelings of guilt that they did not do enough to prevent the
events from occurring. They sometimes have a belief that their life will terminate
prematurely – which is perhaps partly wish fulfillment, but may in some cases be a
realistic assessment of their situation! It is not always easy to rid the sufferer of his
symptoms, particularly of the intrusive ideas. But it is frequently possible to reduce the
degree of distress they cause by a range of therapeutic techniques, which get the sufferer
to reconstruct the vivid details of the past traumatic experiences and to share the feelings
evoked with a sympathetic listener. Such therapy is often found to be most beneficial
when conducted with groups of sufferers who have had similar experiences, since the
individual is enabled to gain reassurance that the troubling experience of intrusive ideas
and the feelings that accompany them are not that unusual. Those who are persistently
troubled by feelings of guilt can also gain relief by group debriefings. This enables them
to gain a sense that the responsibility was not entirely theirs but is to be seen as shared
with others, or that they were caught up in something that was simply inevitable.

For children in Freetown who have served with the fighting forces, it seems that
memories of shocking events are never far beneath the surface. They are in evidence the
moment children are encouraged to draw. In this respect, the difference are striking
between the drawings of children who have been conscripted into the fighting forces, and
those who have been in displaced persons camps. The former children show great
eagerness to explain their drawings of butchery and devastation in minute detail to a
concerned adult: notwithstanding the fact that this may frequently cause them much
distress, they seem to derive much comfort from sharing their experiences with others.
Children also get consolation from listening to and supporting one another in group
sessions. They listen pensively with rapt attention as another child explains her drawing.
They show obvious signs of recognizing one another's experiences, and readily help
another child out with her explanation when the going gets emotionally difficult.

Willingness to listen to what these children have to say about there past unpleasant
experiences does seem important, but it would be a mistake to focus energies too tightly
on this. In contrast to the sufferer from posttraumatic stress disorder, these children do
not experience their memories as distressing and unwanted intrusions into their thinking.
The memories seldom seem to give rise to panic, emotional disorientation, or distraction
from the tasks children have to perform and distract them from other tasks. Rather they
are just part of the child's unpleasant personal history that he goes over time and time
again as he tries to make sense of what has happened to him, and to learn some lessons
for the future. What preoccupies these children much more, and a cause them panic and
distress is thoughts about the dangers of the future. Unfortunately, short of engaging in
gross deceit and lulling them into a sense of false security, there is often little we can do
to calm this panic and distress. If children could be helped to feel more secure about the

future, then perhaps they would be more concerned to leave the past behind. Memories would be experienced as intrusive, unwanted and distressing and intrusive memories would give them much more reason for distress. So long as children find their memories of the past helpful guides for future action, any therapeutic procedure which sought to make these memories less accessible would seem to be counter-indicated; and the frequently heard call that children should be encouraged to forget the past should be resisted.

Another notable difference between these children and the victim of posttraumatic stress disorder lies in their way of viewing guilt. Far from being constantly racked by guilt, the child ex-combatant seems confused about the degree of his responsibility for his actions, and vacillates between describing them as highly heroic and deeply evil. Children do at times show signs of persisting feelings of guilt, but they are more commonly heard to boast about their actions than to express remorse. When children are troubled, it is frequently by the felt lack of any stable moral code by which the rightness or wrongness of actions can be judged. It is as though they are trapped on shifting moral ground, and what appears from the lie of the land to be a correct course of action at one moment changes appearance at the next. Clearly, these children do need help with resolving issues of responsibility and guilt, but the procedures developed for the treatment of victims of post traumatic stress disorder hardly seem the most appropriate. Rather than seeking to relieve the child's sense of guilt, the more frequent need is to help the child confront responsibility for wrong, which he defensively denies. In the case of Ibrahim, the psychosocial worker made the following notes on the desirable approach.

In the context of his particular culture, the worries of Ibrahim regarding the impact of his past actions on the present have their own logic. If one harms another person, there is a risk that it will rebound on you, mostly through the intervention of bad spirits. The fact that the actions were not committed through free will, does not eliminate this risks, but it might make it less probable. This logic has to be respected in the therapeutic interventions with Ibrahim. We will certainly not directly challenge his beliefs that his suffering might be related to his misconduct. We will look at the possibility of his participating in traditional cleansing rituals of his community. The sense of support he would get from his community. At the same time we will try to bring Ibrahim to think about the level of responsibility he can carry for acts which he does not really remember very well and which he did not do, so it seems, entirely out of free will. In this way, we will aim to lower the anxieties resulting form his actions and to break the vicious circle in which he interprets ever-increasing levels of suffering as proof of his misconduct. At the same time we must work to understand better the mystical references Ibrahim makes regarding the things that he saw or sees. If Ibrahim is indeed having flashbacks of the bad experiences he had under the influence of drugs, these uncontrolled intrusions will undoubtedly also be a major source of additional anxiety in turn fuelling his sense of having done wrong the We will explain to him that flashbacks are a normal consequence of the kind of experiences he had under the influence of drugs, that he could take advantage of the presence and the reassurance of a friend during a flashback in order to maintain contact with reality, and that some relaxation techniques can help him remain in control and help him not to panic.

6. CONCLUSION

6.1. The overriding importance of rebuilding trust and self-esteem

Perhaps the greatest danger of concentrating too tightly on traumatic stress disorder is that it leads us to look only at the impact of individual shocking events and ignore the significance of a whole sequence of abusive experiences the children have undergone The problem for these children is not primarily something they have seen, something they have heard, or even something they have done; it is first and foremost the experience of betrayed trust which comes with being forcefully separated from their family, exposed to danger and violence by adults, made to do things that deep inside they sense to be wrong, and finally handed over at demobilization to those who have previously been portrayed as the enemy. All of this generates inside the children a sense of lack of control over their lives and day-to-day actions; it destroys their sense of self worth, impairs their capacity for normal human relationships, and distorts their capacity for clear moral judgment. In the case of Ibrahim, his conviction that spirits are tormenting him for past wrong-doings is closely linked to the forced drug abuse he was subjected to.

Ibrahim worries that the drugs administered by his captors have caused him some permanent head trauma. We can however reassure him that it is not probable that he was submitted to a dose that would cause necrosis. He never complained of amnesia, hemiplegia or of any other neurological symptoms of cerebral necrosis. If the problems of Ibrahim can be explained by a bad experience under the influence of drugs, we can give him some reassurance that he is probably not the victim of an addictive drug. The suffering, the cravings and the withdrawal symptoms typical of drug addicts are seldom in evidence among the young combatants in Sierra Leone. But even if we can reassure Ibrahim that he did not suffer from any physical trauma, we cannot deny that he is very much handicapped by his anxiety attacks and his constant worries. His behavior gets worse every day. If Ibrahim is really using the drugs bought in the village, it is because he is trying to escape from his sufferings. But he also complains of feeling more agitated under the influence of drugs. Can it be that we are looking at the anxiety of someone he sees himself embarked on a course that leads nowhere, because even if drugs can for a while make him forget about the past, it does not change it? Or is it that the drugs he buys at the dealer have the effect of agitating him even more instead of calming him? Whatever the role of the drugs acquired in the village, it is obvious that the problems of Ibrahim will not be resolved as long as we can't get him to deal with his anxieties concerning his experiences and actions in his past. As soon as he can arrive at a more acceptable interpretation of the latter, the temptation to look for relief in drugs will not be the same.

Part of the reason perhaps why destruction of trust is so disturbing to the children is because it puts reason and biology in conflict. John Bowlby – perhaps the greatest authority ever on the emergence of relationships between small children and their caregivers – once pointed out that if the young infant did not have built in at birth a natural tendency to draw the caregiver towards it, or to seek out the protection of the caregiver at moments of danger, he/she would not survive (Cicchety et al., 1993). In these early behaviors we see the origins of a relation of trust that is equally important to older children. The older child who is exposed to physical, emotional or moral danger by adults can learn that such trust is unwise, but the biological tendency which naturally pulls the child back into an unwise relation with the adult is hard to resist at moments when the child feels a strong need for support. At such moments we see strikingly ambivalent patterns of behavior, with the child making an overtures but then pulling back from the relationship, or even rejecting the adult violently as they become aware of the dangers of what they are doing. We also see perplexity and distress as the child tries to make sense of patterns of behavior which are not fully in her control. The professional too feels distress as she reaches out and tries to help the child rebuild trust – only to have her overtures rejected.

Equally challenging is the task of rebuilding the child's sense of self-worth. Low self-esteem is of course a frequent problem of children who have been persistently abused and exploited. Among other things, such children frequently receive the depersonalizing message that they have value only for a particular service – sexual or other – that they can provide here and now. Because they receive praise only for the services they render, and not for what they are and can do, they cease to think of themselves as people with capacities that can be cultivate and use to gain the admiration of others. Sense of worth can hit an all-time low when they are discarded from service because they are no longer needed, and this is why the problem is particularly acute for the child who has recently been demobilized. Already humiliated by their hand-over to the enemy, children who have been released by the fighting forces seem over sensitive to anything that could be taken as a further threat to failing self-esteem. Even well intentioned acts can be interpreted by them as yet another humiliations to which they respond catastrophically with outbursts of rage. The outbursts of rage can be confusing to the child himself, and compound his sense of humiliation through giving him the feeling that he is showing himself to be out of control.

6.2. Helping children with the realities of right and wrong

Such catastrophic behavior can easily frustrate attempts to help children address the rights and wrongs of their past actions. As is the case with other abused children, low self-esteem is frequently compounded by a deep sense of having done things that are wrong or wicked. Generally, this is acknowledged only very reluctantly. Frequently children will boast of what they have done, but it is readily detectable that underneath they have grave misgivings. Their boasting is more aimed at gaining reassurance from their peers that what they did was not all bad, and that it had an element of heroism. It is one way the child has of protecting his self-esteem from total collapse. If we allow ourselves to be provoked into challenging this boasting behavior and exposing the child's actions for what they were, we destroy the child's attempts to bolster his self-esteem, throw him into rage and lose his collaboration.

The psychosocial worker who will do the intervention with Ibrahim should be aware of the presence of anxieties Ibrahim might not be able to express, but which are very important to him and might have a big influence on his behavior. Maybe

*he feels guilty about the death of his parents. Is there a confusion in his head
between the implicit betrayal of deserting his parents at the time of the abduction,
and some imaginary misconduct under the influence of drugs? The spirits that
haunt him as a form of revenge for the things he did under the influence of drugs –
are they being mixed up with the spirits of his parents, who might in his view be
angry because he failed to defend them and also failed to bury them? Only a
sensitivity to all these possibilities would enable the psychosocial worker to give
Ibrahim the necessary reassurance for him to overcome his anxieties.*

Children have various defenses they can bring to protect their self-esteem and avoid
the conclusion that they are all bad when confronted with their guilt, and all of these can
readily stand in the way of helping them to clarify moral issues. They may try to
convince themselves that paradoxically there was some good in what they did; or they
may try to deny to themselves that the action was really their responsibility; or they may
try to repress their sense of guilt and push matters from their mind. If we are to penetrate
these defenses and help children to face up to the moral issues raised by their past
actions, we have first to help them bolster their self-esteem. We have to tread a long road
to help them to identify the truly positive in themselves and in their actions, and to build
up a proper image of the good me so that they no longer need so urgently to deny the bad
they have done. But all the time we have to be aware of just how fragile the child feels,
and how quickly he will defend himself by shutting us out if he feels threatened. We have
to remember too that in a war where children are allied first to one side and then to
another, they grow accustomed to morality being on shifting sands. This makes it all too
easy to engage in defensive denial of having done wrong.

6.3. Creating an Environment of Caring Adults

*We are still far from understanding the problems of Ibrahim. A child who
underwent an abduction, the murder of his parents, drug intoxication, personal
violence and the forced participation in atrocities must have very strong defenses.
He must have very complex worries regarding what he has done and regarding
himself. He must have strong resistances in his human relations. As the
psychosocial worker establishes a closer relationship with Ibrahim, the latter will
gain more confidence in explaining himself. He will be able to think more frankly
about his problems and, we hope, to master them.*

Helping these children to rebuild trust and restore self-esteem can at times seem
daunting because of the children's difficulties in sustaining a relationship with a therapist,
and their worries that any working situation with an adult might expose them as bad and
worthless. Yet it is striking how trust does become restored simply through the children's
day-to-day experience of good care, and how this has a knock on effect for self-esteem.
So strong is the children's biological urge to find adults they can trust that despite their
determination to avoid relationships, they can nevertheless be seen seeking out trial
situations. How frequently do we see a newly arrived child in a reception center for
demobilized children coldly dismissing offers of help from staff, but nevertheless
listening with rapt attention at some distance to adult conversations for some signal that a
trusting relationship is possible. How frequently do we see the same child – still

emotionally distant and reserved – come back some time later to try the adults further with some meager enquiry or request for help. And then the next day we see the same child seeking treatment from the nurse for some phantom pain or ache, and deriving reassurance from the gentle touching. And yet a few days later – after some clearly staged misdemeanor, which results in heavy scolding – we see the same child return to find out whether the adult's care and commitment has the strength to withstand the recent provocation.

This process of reparation, which seems to happen quite naturally when children experience an environment of caring and concerned adults, should give us confidence. If it is possible for us to achieve this with the children in a reception center, there is hope that the same reparation can be achieved in Sierra Leone society at large, since the world of children is in many ways just a microcosm of the larger society, which is also trapped in a mind-set of mistrust. But for those adults who must work with children in reception centers and in their homes to restore mental health, their own mistrust does not make the task an easy one. These people have themselves suffered at the hands of armed groups. Their loved ones have been murdered and their homes burned down – sometimes by the children they must care for. They also experience feelings of bitterness, anger and vindictiveness. When faced with callousness and rejection from children who have done so much destruction, these people are driven all too easily to conclude that the children are evil and beyond any possible help. At these dangerous moments, they see in the children something that must be destroyed, before it is allowed to destroy the rest of society. They speak aggressively of the need to cut behaviors out, or break the child's habits, or knock the child down to size. Children are quick to pick up these destructive feelings and move speedily into defensive mode. In this way a lot of good work on the building of trust and self-esteem can quickly be undone. For the expatriate who works alongside local mental health workers caring for these children in Sierra Leone, the greatest challenge perhaps lies with helping her fellow professionals maintain sensitivity to these dangers: It is helping them to gain deeper insight into the terrible psychological legacy left by a destructive war, and to find the inner resources to contribute more fully to a new future.

REFERENCES

Cicchety, D., Toth, S.L, & Lynch, M. (1993) The developmental sequel of child maltreatment: implications for war trauma. In Leavitt, A.L. & Fox, N. A. (eds.) *The psychological effects of war and violence on children*, 41-71. Hillsdale, NJ: Lawrence Erlbaum.

Garbarino, J. & Kostelny, K. (1993) Children's responses to war: what do we know? In Leavitt, A.L. & Fox, N. A. (eds.), *The psychological effects of war and violence on children*, 23-41. Hillsdale, NJ: Lawrence Erlbaum.

Jareg, E. & Mc Callin, M. (1993) *The rehabilitation of former child soldiers in Sierra Leone*. Geneva: International Catholic Child Bureau.

Parson, E.R. (1996) It takes a village to heal a child. *Journal of Contemporary Psychotherapy 26*, 251-286.

Machel, G. (2001) Child Soldiers. In: *The impact of war on children*; a *review of progress since the 1996 United Nations report on the Impact of Armed Conflict on Children*, 7-25. Geneva: UNICEF.

McConnan, I. & Uppard, S. (2001) *Children - Not Soldiers: Guidelines for working with child soldiers and children associated with fighting forces*. New York: Save the Children.

UNICEF, Coalition to Stop the Use of Child Soldiers (2003) *Guide to the optional protocol on the involvement of children in armed conflict*. Geneva: UNICEF.

Yule, W. & Williams, R. M. (1990) Post-traumatic reactions in children. *Journal of Traumatic Stress 3*, 179-195.

Web sites:
http://www.unicef.org/emerg/index_childsoldiers.html
www.childsoldiers.org

6. "MY WHOLE BODY IS SICK ...
MY LIFE IS NOT GOOD"
A Rwandan asylum seeker attends a
psychiatric clinic in London

Derek Summerfield[1]

Sara was a 32-year-old Rwandan woman who arrived alone in Britain in April 1997. In October 1997, she was referred by her general practitioner (GP) to my psychiatry clinic at the Medical Foundation for the Care of Victims of Torture, a charity offering services to asylum seekers and refugees. The referral letter stated that Sara was evoking considerable concern in her social workers and others, was increasingly depressed, sleepless and had intrusive thoughts. The letter also noted that Sara was a frequent attender at the GP surgery with somatic complaints. An urgent appointment was being sought.

1. BACKGROUND

Before seeing Sara I read the account she had given to her lawyer as the basis for her asylum claim. Born of a Hutu Rwandan father and Ugandan mother in Rwanda, she had completed primary schooling. At the time of the catastrophic events in Rwanda in 1994 (14% of the population – mainly Tutsis but also moderate Hutus – slaughtered in 3 months) she was married to a Hutu Rwandan, with five children aged 5-13 years. In the aftermath, when the largely Tutsi Rwandan Popular Front took over government, her husband left his post as an army sergeant and they devoted themselves to farming their small piece of land.

One day in December 1995, during a meeting in their home in which they and other Hutus were discussing the situation, the door was broken down and soldiers entered. Her husband and the other men scattered. The soldiers beat Sara and her mother to obtain information and then killed both her parents with machetes in front of her. She was taken to an army barracks and acid was poured on parts of her body. She was kept for a month in a mud hut and regularly raped. Then a soldier who had taken pity on her helped her to

---

[1] Derek Summerfield, Institute of Psychiatry, King's College, London

escape with the help of a Catholic priest. Arrangements were made for her to leave the country and she traveled via Nigeria, eventually flying to Britain. Since that day she had had no news of any kind about her husband or children.

This was not the first time that Sara had been referred to the Medical Foundation. In May 1997, a few weeks after her arrival, her social worker made a referral because she was worried by Sara's mental state. The manager of the hostel where she was living saw her as anxious and suspicious, and recorded that Sara said she wanted to walk back to Rwanda. There were concerns about suicide risk. Sara was allocated to a clinical psychologist at the Medical Foundation who found her very distressed but unwilling or unable to talk very much. She was offered a regular appointment but after attending on three occasions Sara dropped out and did not respond to a letter inviting her to resume.

2. THE INTERVIEW

I saw her with an interpreter. She looked subdued or unhappy but composed. From my verbatim notes, the first thing she said to me was: "I'm not depressed, I'm ill". She said her whole body was ill, but particularly her head which could become 'big'. She said she had terrible headaches, could not sleep and could not do anything.

When I asked her what she saw as her number one current problem, she told me it was the hostel: "the place makes me sick". She said she had to share a small room; the building was overheated and there was thieving. When asked about other major current problems, she mentioned her scars. She said she had been ill since 1995. When I asked what she saw as the cause of her illness, she replied that it was all her problems, mumbling something about her children and then tailing off into silence. A moment later she asked if she could be excused for a few minutes and left the room.

When she had not returned after five minutes I went out and found her standing in the corridor. Her demeanor had changed and she was obviously angry. She said she refused to talk any further in front of the interpreter, whom she had decided was a Tutsi. She said she was prepared to continue the interview with the English she had learned since being in Britain. I passed this on to the interpreter and Sara and I continued without her. Sara's command of English was better than I had expected.

Her anger disappeared when the interview resumed. She said to me spontaneously that she was not 'depressed' even though her general practitioner was saying that she was because of the loss of her children. Then she went on to make another allusion to her scars, saying that she had been given some massage the day before; this had felt good and had helped her sleep. She told me she was attending a woman's group and was also going to college to improve her English, though sometimes she did not understand the teacher.

She then made a reference to the antidepressant (Amitriptyline) she had been prescribed by her GP for some months, saying: "I am tired of medicine... they are no good". She went on to refer to the three sessions she had attended with a clinical psychologist several months earlier. She said "talk makes me feel tired" and "the doctor says talk is good but I don't think so" and "talk is not bad if you are well ...". Again she switched back to her scars, telling me of the throbbing pain in them. At this point she briefly mentioned that the Red Cross had been attempting to trace her children, but without success. Then she went on to say "people say I am mad", referring to the hostel staff and commenting that this was because of her allegations about thieving.

The next entry in my notes indicates that at this point she spontaneously mentioned her mother being killed in front of her, and that her mother made eye contact with her as she was being cut up. She said that this memory or image could 'shoot' at her at times: "the way she comes makes me feel bad".

Then she reverted to her current problems, telling me that her very helpful social worker was leaving her job: "who will help me now?" to change to a better hostel. Her last remark in the interview was: "my whole body is sick ...my life is not good".

I did not ask for a systematic account of her experiences, including the rapes and torture (which she did not bring up). As far as mental state was concerned, my conclusions were tempered by my awareness of my limitations. What might a Western psychiatrist authoritatively conclude here? How far did his or her expert writ run? Nonetheless, I did not think she was suicidal, nor that it was useful – or wanted by her – to offer follow-up in a psychiatric clinic. I did not see her again. I heard subsequently that a referral her GP had also made to physiotherapy had been helpful, and that she continued to attend the woman's group regularly.

3. DISCUSSION

3.1. Western psychiatry and non-western distress: common ground, worlds apart or something in between?

In relation to prevailing medical practice in Britain this was not an inappropriate psychiatric referral. Sara brought herself frequently to the GP surgery, could be seen as a case of depression for whom a course of anti-depressants was indicated, and appeared not to be improving. The GP would have known that the social worker and hostel manager were also worried about her. Though the GP's letter did not specifically link the referral to her appalling story, its tone suggested that this was the key factor. This would have as much to do with contemporary social values and assumptions as with medical assessment *per se*. This century has witnessed a spectacular rise in the power of medicine and psychology, displacing religion as the source of explanations and antidotes for the vicissitudes of life. Many experiences far less objectively extreme than those in Sara's story are now expressed in the language of trauma, and viewed as capable of having long-lasting psychological effects (Summerfield, 2001). To many it would seem obvious that Sara needed psychiatric or psychotherapeutic help on this account alone, even if she didn't agree.

For her part Sara did not see herself as an appropriate case for a psychiatrist and indeed her opening statement – "I'm not depressed, I'm ill"- was an explicit reframing from a psychological paradigm to a bodily one. She immediately went on to cite bodily weariness, the sensation that her head and neck had swollen, headaches and poor sleep. Somatic symptoms, which the GP noted Sara had been bringing to the surgery, are the most common clinical expression of distress worldwide. Somatic presentations represent that part of the whole predicament facing a person which he or she thinks is appropriate or expected to bring to a medical setting (Lin et al., 1985).

These are typically deemed 'psychosomatic' in Western medical terminology but this is simplistic. Somatic symptoms are located in multiple systems of meaning serving diverse functions (Kirmayer & Young, 1998). Depending on circumstances they can be seen as:

- an index of disease or disorder (the medical view in Sara's case);
- an indication of particular personality traits;
- a symbolic condensation of intrapsychic conflict;
- a culturally coded expression of distress (likely to apply here, given Sara's background as a Rwandan);
- a medium for expressing social discontent or for a repositioning in a social situation (also likely to apply, given that medicalized presentations may confer advantages for asylum seekers if the doctor is prepared to underwrite their claims for scarce resources like housing).

We can further note that her parting statement – "my whole body is sick..... my life is not good" – is a kind of metaphor for the totality of her experience since 1994. The sick or wounded body she presents stands for her sick or wounded social world, one in which a mother can lose her children and years later still not know if they are alive or dead, in which she and others could be murdered or mutilated with impunity, could lose her role, her place and nation, be cast as a marginal in a distant, strange land.

The additional factor underlying a physical presentation in Sara's case lay in the scar tissue left by the acid burns, associated by her with throbbing pain. Her GP had prescribed painkillers on this account, though Sara saw massage as offering more. The other physical treatment had been the anti-depressants, which both Sara and by implication the GP had seen as ineffective (though it was not unreasonable to have tried them).

The development of psychiatry as a scientific endeavor has its roots in the Enlightenment and in Cartesian assumptions that the inner world of the mind occupies a realm separable from the outer world of the body, and is available for study in a comparable way. With this came an assertion of the causal nature of psychological events and a reliance on positivism to guide theory and research on the singular human being as basic unit of study. All this constitutes an achievement, an ineffably Western one, but not a discovery. There are many true descriptions of the world and what might be called psychological knowledge is the product of a particular culture at a particular point in its history. Western psychiatry is one among many ethnomedical systems, yet it has tended to naturalize its own cultural distinctions, objectify them through empirical data and then reify them as universal natural science categories (Littlewood, 1990). Elsewhere, not least in Rwanda, illness is not conceived of as situated in body or mind alone and taxonomies may draw on physical, supernatural and moral realms in ways totally alien to a Western citizen. Distress or disease is commonly understood in terms of disruptions to the social and moral order, which includes the influences of ancestors and spirits, and internal emotional factors per se are not viewed as capable of being pathogenic. This is not of course to say that 'culture' is homogenous, and that all Rwandans have the same constructions of distress and disorder because they are Rwandans: diversity also arises in relation to education, social class, urban versus rural location, for example.

The lack of fit between Western mental health services and those of non-Western asylum seekers, so evident to both Sara and myself during our interview, is exemplified by the assumptions of the Western trauma discourse. Its flagship is post-traumatic stress disorder (PTSD), an official psychiatry category since 1980. It is perhaps unusual that Sara's referral letter did not mention PTSD, since this has come to be used as a catch-all diagnosis and signifier of the mental state and well-being of survivors of extreme events anywhere. It has become the organizing concept for a fashionable plethora of assistance programs for war-affected peoples, including asylum seekers and refugees in Western Europe. I and others have critiqued and criticized these developments at length elsewhere (Summerfield, 1999a; Bracken, 1998). PTSD may be seen as a Western culture-bound syndrome.

The assumption underpinning such work, one which Sara was in effect holding out against, is that the biopsychomedical paradigm on which Western psychiatry and psychotherapy is based is universally applicable, whether or not recipients see it like this. There is little evidence that war-affected peoples have asked for such interventions, but Western experts are implicitly saying that they know better what war has done to them and what they need. Psychiatric universalism risks being imperialistic, reminding us of the colonial era when what was presented to indigenous peoples was that there were different types of knowledge, and that theirs were second-rate. The notion that 'traumatic stress' causes psychological disruption may be invalid in cultures that emphasize fate, determinism and spiritual influences. There is a serious possibility that the Western trauma discourse imported into the lives of people whose meaning systems have been devitalized by war and forced displacement might impair their struggle to reconstitute a sense of reality, morality and dignity. After all, the trauma discourse introduces elements that are not mere surface phenomena but core components of Western culture: a theory of human development and identity, a secular source of moral authority, a sense of time and a theory of memory (Argenti-Pillen, 2000).

Taussig (1980), while applauding the emphasis which the new cross-cultural psychiatry gave to elucidating the patient's model of illness, nonetheless cautioned that the knowledge so obtained could allow the management of the patient to be all the more persuasive or coercive. Said (1993) notes that a salient trait of modern imperialism is that it claims to be an education movement, setting out consciously to modernize, develop, instruct and civilize, echoing the earlier writings of such as Cesaire and Fanon on the surreptitious incorporation of the ideologies of colonial dependence and racial inferiority into modern psychological discourse.

It is a category fallacy to assume that because PTSD features can apparently be identified worldwide, they mean the same thing everywhere (Kleinman, 1987). In practice, since PTSD criteria distinguish poorly between the physiology of normal distress and the physiology of pathological distress, over-recruitment of cases is typical. The most graphic, recent example of this was a community survey of 245 randomly selected, non-helpseeking adults in war-torn Freetown, Sierra Leone, in which PTSD was ascribed to 99% (de Jong et al., 2000). In these circumstances PTSD is a pseudocondition.

There is little doubt that Sara was diagnosable as a case of PTSD, though I did not choose to do this. In particular, proponents of trauma work would light on the image she carried of her mother's murder, able to distressingly 'shoot' at her, as evidence of the 'traumatic' memory often conceptualized as the core of the disorder. The backdrop to this, as Hacking (1995) argues, is that as scientific understandings of ourselves have come to replace religious ones, the notion of 'soul' has been supplanted by a focus on memory – to be seen as a thing open to scientific enquiry. The problem is that memory is fluid, variegated, untidy, inconsistent and indeed contradictory. There is no unearthing of the past in pristine condition, no one definitive narrative. A search for the meaning of something, whether a specific calamity or, say, the realization that one's life is generally unhappy, may drive a different scanning of the past than if one was not impelled to such a search: the act of remembering is interpretative. Memory is in interplay between private and public realms, addresses social as much as personal identity, and is thus shaped by the context in which the telling takes place and the purpose to which it is to be put. It may have as much to do with the future, via the wish to give this a particular shape, as the past. This understanding of memory is familiar to anthropology, though regrettably not to psychiatry, and is a principal point of departure between the two disciplines (Foxen, 2000; Summerfield, 2000; Skultans, 1998). It might be asked why psychiatric science and practice has been so impervious to insights from anthropology.

When Gulf War ex-soldiers were asked a standard set of questions tapping their combat experiences one month after the war, and again two years later, significant discrepancies emerged: the second account tended to report more traumatic exposure than the first (Southwick et al., 1997). (This shift may well be pertinent to the construction of so-called Gulf War Syndrome, which is still seeking the disease status accorded PTSD). Civilian accounts of war will have victim, protagonist (and sometimes perpetrator) themes intertwined. Sara would not tell quite the same story in quite the same way to an aid worker in Rwanda, to a doctor in London, a British immigration official, a human rights tribunal, or fellow asylum seekers. If I had been a Rwandan language speaker, her presentation to me that day in my clinic could not have been exactly the same.

Traumatic memory is a psychiatric construct rather than natural entity (Young, 1995). There have always been painful and disturbing recollections, and it would be strange if Sara did not still have these. However, the reification of traumatic memory - a private, static, circumscribed, universal and pathological entity which reveals itself in flashbacks and re-experiencing and requires processing – is in general a caricature of reality.

In her very first remark in the interview Sara, referred to depression. The following problems bedevil any claim that depression might have to be a universally valid construct: the cross-cultural variations in the definition of selfhood (and of human nature); differing local categories of emotions; the difficulty of translating emotion- related vocabulary because of cultural variations in language use; the absence of a biological marker (Marsella & White, 1982; Littlewood, 1990). Even in the West the term is used very variably, and often figuratively. Even if Sara had agreed with her GP that she had depression, it would not be because the term had a precise equivalent in Rwandan culture. Rather, it would be because she realized that this was part of the lexicon of distress in the new society, and one legitimated by doctors. At a time when they have few allies of their own, asylum seekers see it as in their interests to present in ways that are intelligible, and if possible compelling, to the medical gaze. Indeed asylum seekers may pick up that terms like nightmares or flashbacks have a certain currency in relation to the traumatic account on which their asylum application depends, and use them accordingly. Thus the imperatives of asylum-seeking independently influence what is brought to medical settings, the way a story is told and the words chosen to illuminate it.

It is because medicalized and psychologized thinking is now so embedded in popular constructions of common sense, and in the aesthetics of expression, that not to automatically use the language of trauma can make it seem that the horrific nature of Sara's experiences is being played down. There is little doubt that Sara is an unhappy, haunted woman, and in part she does see herself as dysfunctional. The question is what grip

Western psychiatry and its methods can have on her predicament. As far as treatment is concerned, it is mainstream mental health services that will be on offer in Western countries of asylum, for better or worse, though I suggest that their grip can only be a limited one. As far as documentation is concerned, the medicopsychiatric consequences of extreme experiences may be part of a counting of costs (and generate a report for asylum-seeking purposes), yet it is only a narrowly instrumental style of reasoning that suggests that torture and atrocity are a bad thing because PTSD is diagnosable in victims. Indeed the diagnosis cannot distinguish between past torture or a bicycle accident, nor exclude pre-existing psychiatric problems, nor the impact of current social difficulties.

For the record, during the 1990s I personally assessed over 800 asylum seeker or refugee survivors of organized violence and persecution selectively referred because of concerns (sometimes their own) held to warrant a psychiatric opinion. I saw plenty of unhappiness, frustration, anger and humiliation but the overwhelming majority of these people were not ill, by which I mean they had no significant breakdown in their capacity to function adaptively and to manage their lives. We must realize the limitations of a discourse in which the effects of state violence and atrocity are represented as individual illness and vulnerability. As Zarowsky (2000) puts it, this discourse may erase the very experience of coercion, powerlessness and threat - and the variety of human responses to these - that attention to the human costs of war promises. We need a greater responsibility to acknowledge Otherness.

3.2. Meaning, morality, talk therapy and healing

Collectively held beliefs about the consequences of highly negative experiences carry an element of self-fulfilling prophecy in their capacity to influence individual victims, shaping what they feel has been done to them, whether or how they seek help, and their expectations of recovery. In the clinical setting the mental health professional is part of this process, shaping the very words victims come to use to describe themselves and the legacy of their histories. The rise of talk therapies and counseling to address ever greater areas of life has been a significant trend in Western societies in the past two generations. It rests on a particular view of a person, a moral view, as an autonomous individual, a mini-universe of emotions, aspirations, conflicts etc., who is capable of changing him or herself in isolation from social context. The best candidates for talk therapy are often said to be psychologically minded, having a Western viewpoint and indeed a middle-class Western viewpoint. A core assertion, and this runs through the whole trauma field, is that distress or suffering is detachable from those carrying it and is a circumscribed technical problem amenable to mental health technologies.

In practice, talk therapy represents a kind of social movement, and in many respects an industry, and has not relied on rigorous theorizing and evidence-based practice. Little valid research has been done, though two recent studies of one-off trauma counseling have cast doubt on its efficacy and suggested that harm can be done if clients pick up the idea that they should ruminate on what happened and not put it aside (Wessely et al., 1998; Mayou et al., 2000; Kenardy, 2000).

Nonetheless, the assumption that professionally guided emotional catharsis or working through is universally valid and necessary for war victims has gained considerable currency. In USA and Europe a number of specialist centers have been operating for victims of torture, in particular, and this interview took place in one. The tendency has been to pitch the psychological impact of experiences like Sara's as having a special nature and demanding special expertise, not just in treatment but also in documentation for asylum-seeking purposes. But the testimony of experts is powerful only to the extent that their expertise is real. If asylum seekers like Sara are not understood to have a characteristic and distinct form of mental state (and they don't have), then the testimony of sympathetic professionals is simply that: sympathetic. Further, the claim – to be seen in the publicity literature of such centers – that people like Sara are likely to have a deep, potentially long term psychological wound requiring expert intervention (though a few may see themselves like this), casts them as a damaged and diminished group for whom others (the center staff) should speak. To effectively equate human pain with impairment can do war victims a far-reaching disservice, since it may muffle what they themselves want to say (not least politically), distort assistance priorities, and color how society comes to think of them, and they of themselves.

A recent example was the confidential recommendation made by the British Home Office strategy group handling the reception of 4,000 Kosovan refugees being airlifted to Britain in mid-1999. Writing at a point when most had not even landed, they nonetheless stated that the Kosovans were "in a serious state of trauma and chronic illness with a need for long term counseling and support" (Guardian, 1999). But a subsequent study of a large number of these refugees painted a very different picture. Very few saw themselves as having a mental health problem at all, let alone a long-term one, bearing out observations by refugee workers that there had been no demand for counseling (N. Savage, personal communication). So who knew best?

The intention is not to cast Western and non-Western cultures as two monolithic blocs and the Kosovans are after all white Europeans. But for non-Western asylum seekers in particular, the very idea of the detached introspection of emotions, professionally guided, is alien. Indeed, one problem is that the cultural worlds in which people are immersed can differ so dramatically that translation of emotional terms needs more than merely finding semantic equivalents. Describing how it feels to be grieving or melancholy in another society draws one into an analysis of radically different ways of being a person (Kleinman and Good, 1985). In her study of Somali refugees in Ethiopia, Zarowsky (2000) noted that emotional experience and expression were interpreted primarily with respect to what they indicated about sociopolitical, not intrapsychic, processes. It was not that Somalis could not psychologize, but that the organizing framework reflected a context in which survival was the overriding concern.

> In many cultures the harmony of the family or group matters more than the autonomy of the individual, who is not conceived of as a freestanding unit. Thus, containment of emotion and adaptation to social circumstances are viewed as signs of maturity. Fostering individualism through talk therapy may put people at odds with their families or local worlds (Kirmayer & Young, 1998).

Sara was referred twice to the Medical Foundation by a caring GP who had concerns about her current mental state, but was doubtless also horrified by her story. It is the caring Western citizen as much as the caring doctor who would feel that surely a woman who had lost 5 children, been multiply raped and witnessed grotesque atrocities directed at her parents, needed be assessed by a mental health professional, and to talk it through.

The first referral led to sessions with a psychologist, which Sara broke off prematurely. The GP had acted in good faith but clearly Sara had felt coerced: "The doctor says talk is good but I don't think so". The three sessions with the psychologist had not persuaded her that this was a relevant activity – "talk makes me feel tired" – though she added (perhaps a conciliatory gesture to those she knew were trying to help), "talk is not bad if you are well..." The question also begged here is what constitutes informed consent when asylum seekers have so little social clout.

This insistence on a need for counseling, however it might strike recipients, has a wider Rwandan perspective: the establishment of the National Trauma Program and Center in Kigali, sponsored by UNICEF, after the events of 1994. By 1996 over 6,000 trauma advisors were reported to have received training (from outsiders), and 144,000 children had been contacted. Did ordinary Rwandans ask for this, given their pressing post-war problems, and given that trauma and counseling were entirely foreign concepts? It is instructive to transpose this situation to the Jewish Holocaust. A project, planned from afar and using a foreign psychology and its practices, is mobilized in 1945 to address concentration camp survivors. The project leaders have not worked in the area before and know little of its history and culture. The project is funded, say, for one year, the objective being to purge subjects of the trauma of the Holocaust. Such an endeavor would surely be self-evidently presumptuous and unethical.

Some asylum seekers and refugees do make creative attempts to engage with this kind of work and, at a time when they have few other influential allies, may become attached to their therapists. One exception to the general paucity of research was an evaluation of therapeutic work given to asylum seekers in the Netherlands by local therapists. Though both therapists and patients gave an optimistic account of the sessions, marked differences in culturally and situationally determined expectations were evident. Therapists placed primary emphasis on the subjective psychological world of their clients, and on PTSD, and saw culture and the social problems all asylum seekers face, as issues outside the room. The patients spoke positively of the therapists, albeit sometimes seeing them as rather detached. They expressed surprise that therapists had paid so much attention to their childhood and said they had hoped for more practical help (Boomstra & Kramer, 1997; see also Chapter 8). In a recent survey of asylum seekers in London, 76% of those offered counseling or psychotherapy rated it as poor or very poor (Baluchi, 1999). In the mental health clinic refugees may naturally appreciate an empathic, non-judgmental listener but this is a non-specific benefit. (Indeed it might be argued that the mental health sciences have co-opted these and other facets of ordinary human solidarity and fraternity, mystifying them into technical procedures which require experts). The question here, and not just with asylum seekers and refugees, is whether benefits may accrue from talk therapy which are specific to a particular methodology and underlying theory.

Talk therapy has historical roots in Stoic ideas and, later, in Judeo-Christian traditions of confession, forgiveness and of turning the other cheek. It aims to change not just behavior but mind, the way a person construes. It trades on an ethos of acceptance: it is the person, not society that is meant to change (Ingleby, 1989). One reflection of this may be how uncomfortable the clinic or clinician can be when the client or patient forcefully expresses anger, that most moral of emotions. Expressions of grief or sadness are seen as the stuff of clinic work, but anger is difficult. It has been noted that in successful therapy the worldview of the client moves closer to that of the therapist. What does it mean to people like Sara that in one sense therapy is a form of persuasion? What does it mean that she sits opposite a professional who has not in fact experienced atrocity or grotesque loss, but who may have the power to define what it has done to her and what she needs to do to recover? Whose words will count at this critical moment in her life?

Mental health work, and the settings in which this is delivered, are traditionally regarded as politically and morally neutral. Yet the distress which war victims bring into the room points outwards at the political environment which evoked it. An apolitical humanitarianism cannot make full sense to them, even if there are gains in the short term. They are in no doubt that political questions are at the heart of what has happened to them, and what needs to be done. For her part Sara gave me a sharp reminder that she did not regard herself as in a neutral space when she interrupted the interview and left the room angrily. She objected to a Tutsi Rwandan interpreter because the soldiers who had attacked her and her family were, I presumed, Tutsi – but perhaps there was a more general political reason too. Rwandan society and politics was right there with us in the clinic.

For the therapist, acceptance, coming to terms with the past, or processing may be synonyms for healing – the purpose of therapy. But victims may have to struggle with whether acceptance is merely a marker of their impotence and humiliation or, worse still, an acquiescence in injustice – on their part, by those they know and by the Western -led world order which behind the rhetorical screen of human rights retains the *realpolitik* of business as usual. The rise of programs offering talk therapy is certainly sometimes seen cynically by those for whom they are intended, experienced as patronizing or indeed a kind of pacification. In Bosnia, people derisively referred to the model of aid delivered to them as 'bread and counseling', a model which did not offer physical protection, restitution or justice.

A number of these programs has sought to address brutalization, by which an unforgiving (traumatized) victim is held to turn into a potential perpetrator (as a form of mental ill-health) and perpetuate what is called the cycle of violence. Rwanda and former Yugoslavia have particularly attracted facile analyses of this kind and, for example, a foreign-funded project sought to counsel war-affected Croatian children not to hate and mistrust Serbs. Should Sara be counseled not to hate Tutsis, for the sake of her own health and that of her nation, particularly after the anger she revealed for the Tutsi interpreter? Indeed, should Jewish survivors of Nazi genocide have been counseled in the 1940's not to hate Germans? The framing of some current research is illustrative of this medicalization of what was previously a religious piety, the quietist Christian values mentioned already – particularly forgiveness and turning the other cheek. (It is what Bacon in the seventeenth century expressed as: 'he who planneth revenge keeps his own wounds green, which otherwise would heal and do well'). In a recently published study of survivors of apartheid era human rights abuses in South Africa, some of whom testified to the Truth and Reconciliation Commission, PTSD and depression were said to be significantly higher in those who were unforgiving towards the perpetrators, compared to those with high forgiveness scores (Kaminer et al., 2001). The authors did not claim that the lack of forgiveness was necessarily causal rather than correlative, but such studies are seeking to consolidate the notion that it is bad for the mental health of victims if they do not forgive.[2]

Similarly, a survey of 600 Kosovo Albanian households by the Centers for Disease Control and Prevention (1999) found that 86% of men and 89% of women had strong feelings of hatred towards their Serbian oppressors. 51% of men and 43% of women said they had a desire to seek revenge most or all of the time. The title of the survey, as well as methodology and use of psychological instruments, made it explicit that these sentiments were to be cast as mental (ill)-health phenomena. But one man's revenge is another's social justice. The question is whether anger, hatred and a felt need for revenge in those grievously wronged are a bad thing. Don't they carry a moral interrogative (again, the Why), pointing to a social wound as well as to an individual one, and to shared ideas about justice, accountability and punishment which hold a social fabric together? Don't they demand answers? Were the Nuremburg trials of Nazi war leaders after World War 2, which handed down capital punishment in many cases, the result of brutalization, of unhealthy feelings of hatred and revenge in traumatized victims of Nazism? Or did the trial provide a demonstration of justice in action, thus assisting a sense of closure after man-made catastrophe?

Refugee stories are moral tales. "We are not mad, we are betrayed" was the response of one refugee approached by a pilot Bosnian mental health project in Britain (McAfee, 1998). This response is witness to the collectivity (We) of the experience of war and refugeedom, and poses a fundamental question: 'are we impaired or wronged?' If both, how does the mental health profession frame the relationship between the two? How does the psychiatrist or psychotherapist trained to deliver technical outputs see the question of moral knowledge. This is the kind of knowledge that springs from a crisis (a serious accident, a diagnosis of cancer, a social upheaval) which shakes up an individual's assumptions about the world, his or her personal values and priorities. For the war victim, this invokes some of the most urgent questions of the day: the man made demolition of worlds, the impunity of the perpetrators, the indifference of the world order, the near possibility of restoring what was there before. These are Why? or Why me? questions, addressing a moral domain. Medical science is good at How? questions, which are technical ones, but only addresses the Why? by reference to impersonal statistics and epidemiology. The patient may be alone with his anxiety to locate the social and moral meaning of the crisis (Taussig, 1980).

The professional is not of course personally immune to a sense of moral outrage. An especially horrific or poignant story often induces in workers a particular identification with the person concerned, with extra energy devoted to treatment and advocacy. Part of this is the impulse to charity, in the Christian tradition springing from a sense of pity (and Sara may well see herself as pitiable). This works best when its object can be viewed as worthy victim pure and simple, shorn of complexity and context. Understandably, asylum seekers stories seek to deliver up their central character or characters in this form, sometimes with exaggeration or fabrication. The story is in many respects an artefact,

---

[2] Their other finding was that giving testimony to the Truth and Reconciliation Commission did not alter psychiatric status or attitudes to forgiveness (though, from other sources, many of those who did testify were reportedly pleased that they had had the opportunity to do so). It is also indicative of the implicit moral framework that the Commission was not uncomfortable if testifiers wept while giving evidence, but did not like them to become angry. In this study 'recovery' was defined mechanistically and medically, and the psychiatric instruments and categories used were of questionable validity for this population.

constructed for a particular climate of asylum-seeking and help-seeking, and it is no surprise that it can sometimes seem rather formulaic. But it begs to be believed and indeed must be, more or less unreservedly, if the moral impulse to help is not to be diluted. But once some apparently implausible element is noticed and can't be rationalized, a taint may be cast on the integrity of the whole. The story is the strongest thing an asylum seeker as claimant possesses. When it loses its power, the asylum seeker may in effect be recategorized from deserving to undeserving poor – to recall the way the Victorians approached charity. This can even contaminate the way health-related concerns are appraised, a reminder that mental health practice is impressionistic and loses its bearings if what the patient says (often all there is to go on) is not automatically believed. The clinician may be possessed by a sense of moral and clinical immobilization.[3]

The thrall in which Sara's story might be said to hold me, as with her GP and social worker, began before I even met her, when I was reading it through before the interview. Then I ushered her into my office and as I sat down opposite her, torture, rape and lost children lay in the space between us. The fantasies that possessed me at this moment, before Sara had even opened her mouth, were wholly my own, built on the imagined insertion of myself and people close to me, notably my own child, into such scenes (for this is what the hearer or reader does). The language of my thoughts could only draw on the words, and the hinterlands the words brought with them, familiar to me as a Western culture-carrier, and also as a health professional. Were I to feel that I couldn't be in my right mind after such experiences, or at least a deeply changed person, I would be likely to impute this to Sara – and unavoidably on my terms and in my language. As the interview began, did I unwittingly scan her face for signs of what she had passed through? If signs were there I was not in a position to read them, for the face she maintained (except in her brief reaction to the interpreter) was one of composure and dignity. What might this absence of overt distress denote? In some quarters it might be taken to cast doubt on her credibility: I've certainly heard refugee workers say that they find tears a more authentic expression of what someone has been through than their absence, and tearful clients may be prioritized for assistance. This seems to reflect the emotional expressiveness now taken to be the norm in the West: it is not only what an individual can do, but what he or she should do after a tragedy –partly a matter of aesthetics and partly the belief that to hold one's emotions in is bad for you. In fact Sara's demeanor may reflect the face she deems to be appropriate to bring to interviews with officialdom, including doctors, whether by virtue of background norms or simply her personal style.

I have no reason to doubt the veracity of Sara's story as she has told it, but it cannot be the full story: what it explains, what it might foretell of her future life, is not clear (nor

---

[3] Another source of this immobilization is when the health professional is not politically neutral, and has a different view of the conflict than that conveyed explicitly or implicitly by the asylum seeker's story. For instance, a case was referred to me of a (white) South African wanted for trial on charges involving terrorism and politically inspired murder during the apartheid era. He was seeking a medically attested defense against extradition on the grounds that he had PTSD. I refused to see him, and felt he should be extradited. It might also apply, more subtly, to a Bosnian Serb asylum seeker whose version of events seemed at odds with the generally held conclusion that far fewer Serbs were victims, and far more were aggressors, than were Bosnian Muslims. Of course it might similarly be said that few Hutus were victims by comparison with Tutsis, but for me this did not intrude on Sara's case. Lastly, there is the situation faced by a college student counselor in London who opened the newspaper to discover that the nice young Rwandan in whose welfare she was taking considerable interest had just been indicted as a local organizer of the mass killings in 1994.

definitively to Sara at this point). Firstly, how much can I know of what her experiences really mean to her (and it is meaning that matters)? As a Hutu woman and mother what did she think and do during the 3 months of slaughter in 1994, with Hutus massacring Tutsi men, women and children, and also moderate Hutus who opposed the persecution. What role did Sara's husband play, a Hutu soldier? Though Hutu men did most of the actual killing, Hutu women and children were also active participants, joining machete-wielding mobs besieging places of refuge like churches, hostels and hospitals, denouncing their Tutsi neighbors, and stripping clothing and jewelry from the bodies of the just slain and barely living (African Rights, 1995). Others would have been bystanders, not joining in but not protesting or offering hiding places to Tutsi neighbors either. Some Hutus did hide Tutsis they knew.

But the story would need to go back further than 1994. What version of Hutu identity, and its relation to wider Rwandan citizenship, might Sara have inherited from her parents and immediate community? What version of the social memory of the inter-ethnic massacres of recent decades (1994 was not unprecedented, as the international community tended to assume) was she carrying? What was her understanding of the way that people had made sense of their losses after those disasters, negotiated issues of responsibility, culpability and restitution, repaired family, community and wider societal fabric? A public process of this kind is typically pragmatic, for the past must be squared with the urgent demands of the present. After civil war the supposedly stark categories of victim and perpetrator (in the lexicon of international human rights) are often insufficiently nuanced to be straightforwardly useful to those at the grassroots. As far as 1994 and its still evolving legacy is concerned, even in London, Sara would have a sense of the conversations flowing between ordinary people back home, going on around the tasks of everyday life, a kind of national stocktaking distilling through the micro-worlds of individual understanding and experience. This is how people adjust and re-group.

How does Sara connect the 1994 catastrophe to her own horrors of the following year at the hands of soldiers I presume to have been Tutsi? What is her attribution for these horrors, and does any part of their moral charge point inwards as well as outwards? Does she perhaps see what happened to her as a form of punishment at the hands of the wronged? If so, might she feel that she has paid enough, and the debt thus cleared, or is this kind of closure a ridiculous idea to her? What does her reaction to my Tutsi interpreter denote as to her mind set, and how much is she handicapped by being unable to be party to the whole process back home? What has stopped her from returning to Rwanda to search personally for her children?

In the light of all this, what explanatory power should be imputed to a cognitivist model which sees the human mind as the locus of the trauma, and of recovery or healing? This is a mechanistic view of man. Meaning and understanding are seen as stored in the brain in the form of schemata, with questions of morality and responsibility formulated in terms of the sciences of individual psychology and memory. It would carry us rather further into Sara's reality to see meaning as something generated through practical engagement with the world, through a lived life with all its complexity and capacity for multiple interpretations. These are not mere secondary influences, as a trauma model asserts, but the very stuff of a background intelligibility against which her experiences of war and refugeedom are set (Bracken, 2000). It would be a wiser and truer use of the term psychology to define this as an expression of this background intelligibility: a system of thought and practice based on the day-to-day behavior and points of view of the members of a particular group or people. Human misery is a slippery thing, sitting in socio-moral and philosophical domains which themselves are variable and slippery. Nowhere is it straightforwardly subject to processing via a technical intervention in isolation from other aspects of life.

One of the lessons of history may be that the victims of terrible events have largely had to put aside what has happened to them, seek creative accommodation with their altered circumstances and get on with life. It might be said that the imperatives of survival left little choice. Notions of healing, reparation and justice after war have a long history, varying between cultures and over time, though the contemporary discourse of human rights, legalistic and individualistic, is of recent origin. People have always mourned and honored the dead by those means available and familiar to them, with religious or super-natural beliefs and practices typically central. The wider socialization and commemora-tion of grief and loss may be complicated when, as in Rwanda and in 90% of all modern war, the conflict is internal rather than transnational: a winner social group may take over the assets of the losers. Moreover the effects of war cannot be neatly separated off from those of other forces: poverty, landlessness and other forms of structural marginalization, and forced exile. Is the suffering of the world's hungry and undernourished children less of a trauma than that occasioned by bombs and bullets? Recent developments – Truth commissions, international human rights legislation, war crimes tribunals in extended sitting (notably in Bosnia and Rwanda) – do seem promising and are welcomed by some (though not all) victim groups, though their longer term impact remains to be traced (Summerfield, 1997).

Memory is a contemporary Western cultural preoccupation but there is also a need for silence about the past, a line drawn under humiliation. This is not forgetting, but reticence and a conserving of energies (Last, 2000). This kind of silence is not the same as the silence which is a survival strategy in societies where state oppression is pitiless and pervasive. People resume, largely out of sight of helping agencies, the rhythms of every-day life and through banal and unspectacular activities may move towards a sense of normality (albeit not the same normality as before): doing the washing up, taking children to school, helping a neighbor, supporting a football team. They seek to re-establish secu-rity and identity, and for asylum seekers in Europe a point of reference is naturally wage earning (see below). People endure, if only because they must. What personal costs they pay along the way are, with few exceptions, played out in their private lives and not in a mental health clinic. The work of historians, journalists, novelists, poets suggests that there are many who carry the fruits of bitter experience to the grave, and many more- if not most- who could aver to some sense of change in themselves or their attitudes. Not all of this change is negative. Lastly, if a trauma-based view seems to emphasize victims rather than survivors, we should also remember Levi (1988) in *The Drowned and the Saved*, reminding us that the public record is denuded of the accounts of the Drowned.

The observations in the paragraph above are not expert, do not constitute psychiatric insights, are merely the assessment of an ordinary citizen (and one who has not gone through these things). It is for the actors and their historians to say when getting over it or recovery or healing might represent something material, and when merely an abstraction that does little justice to the complexity of what they have passed through.

4. ASYLUM SEEKER REALITIES: REPAIRING A BROKEN SOCIAL WORLD

Two adversarially opposed constructions have predominated in relation to the 4.2 million who have sought asylum in Western Europe in the past decade. Governments, and the conservative social sectors, stress the prevalence of bogus applications by people who are essentially economic migrants. They paint asylum seekers as resilient and wily (rather as they did in the colonial era). Overall this portrayal is too bad to be true. On the other side are the agencies and interests who support asylum seekers, and the liberal and radical social sectors. They pitch asylum seekers as people who had no choice but to run from their countries, innocent of any thought other than to escape further persecution, torture and the risk of death. They do not conjure up resilience, but vulnerability, weakness and damage. This portrayal is too good to be true. The reality, I suggest, is the muddied, uneven, contested ground that lies between the two entrenched positions.

Helping agencies may propagate the second of the images above (often as the traumatized), but their institutional interests sometimes push them to play also to stereotypes like dependent or even manipulative. These can be a self-fulfilling prophecy: agencies see what they expect to see (or what funders want to see), not least because their clients will organize their presentations to fit in with what is on offer at a time of limited options (Harrell Bond, 1999).

A central concern of this paper has been to review the consequences of a medicalized idiom applied too indiscriminately to this population, even as we acknowledge that the medicalization of life has been a major cultural trend across Western societies in this century. This may reduce still evolving experiences, meanings and priorities of asylum seekers from war zones to a single category – trauma – so that refugee suffering is too routinely attributed to pre-flight events, neglecting current factors. There may be risks that the host society offers refugees a sick role rather than what is really sought: opportunities for meaningful citizenship as part of rebuilding a way of life. Sara felt that her body was ill or sick, but she was not seeking the legitimated inactivity and convalescence of a sick role. She was actively seeking more suitable housing, which included her anticipating what else would need to be done once her social worker left her post. She was regularly convening with other women in her situation, an opportunity to acquire useful knowledge and tips on coping in London. She was learning English in college, successfully it seemed to me, a crucial skill in her new setting. Arguably psychiatric models have never sufficiently acknowledged the role of social agency and engagement in promoting mental health.

A Somali asylum seeker, referred for a psychiatric opinion, once said to me with exquisite politeness: "Your words are very fine, doctor, but when are you going to start to help me". Helping agencies have a duty to recognize distress, but then to attend to what the people carrying the distress want to signal by it. Whilst asylum seekers and refugees no doubt bring all that they have been through into the room, as experience embodied, Sara was entirely typical in her focus on practical assistance and advocacy to help bolster her immediate social situation. Housing issues are always a prominent concern. One study of Somali asylum seekers in London showed that insecure housing, not war experiences, torture or death of relatives, was the most significant variable predicting those who would report mental health problems (Dahoud & Pelosi, 1989). So too the question of family reunion, and Sara had sought out the Red Cross because they can help trace missing family members. She may have mentioned it in the interview with me because she thought that my presumed influence as a doctor could add weight to this search.

A service labeled counseling might thus be most acceptable to the majority when it centers on practical problems and directs attention to function-focused and problem-focused coping styles (How are you doing? and What do you need to do?) rather than the emotion-focus (How are you feeling?) more typically associated with counseling and with a Western (but not generally a non-Western) cultural idiom.

Socio-economic and socio-cultural factors are surely key determinants of longer term outcomes. The refugee literature highlights the pivotal role of family and social networks in exile. In Iraqi asylum seekers in London, poor social support was more closely related to low mood or depression than was a history of torture (Gorst-Unsworth & Goldenberg, 1998). In the survey of Kosovan refugees mentioned above, almost everyone nominated work, schooling and family reunion as their major priorities. Work has always been central to the way that newcomers – whether asylum seekers or other category of migrant –established a viable place in the new society, and unemployment levels in Western European countries since the early 1980's have made this a more fraught route than it once was. In the native British population at any rate, unemployment is associated with early death, divorce, family violence, accidents, suicide, higher mortality rates in spouse and children, anxiety and depression, disturbed sleep patterns and low self-esteem (Smith, 1992). There may also be analogies in research in Britain and USA which indicates that those with poor social capital, the poor and socially underconnected, live less long (Wilkinson, 1996; Kawachi & Kennedy, 1997). Women with young children in the lowest fifth of distribution of household income (where asylum seeker families congregate) were at substantially higher risk of poor health and depression. The risk increased further in US states with the biggest differences in incomes between those at the top and those at the bottom (Kahn et al., 2000). The macro- and microfactors mediating such outcomes are complex and still poorly elucidated.

Will some of these trends turn out to be extrapolatable to refugees? Steen's (1993) study of Sri Lankan Tamils compared outcomes in Denmark and Britain. She found that Tamils in Denmark had been effectively deskilled by the extended orientation program provided; even those who had arrived with employable skills had been discouraged by social workers from seeking work until they learnt Danish. In Britain, in contrast, with its *laisser faire* welfare approach, Tamil asylum seekers had an incentive to be independent and economically active as quickly as possible, and were doing much better in coming to terms with their new reality. A recent study in Sweden compared two cohorts of families of survivors of a particular Bosnian concentration camp. The families were originally from the same town in Bosnia and had similar socioeconomic backgrounds. By chance half the families had been sent to a place where there was temporary employment but no psychological services, the other half to a place where no employment was available but there was a full range of psychological services. At follow-up at one year a clear difference had already emerged. The group given work seemed to be doing better, and the majority of adults in the second group were on indefinite sick leave (Eastmond, 1998).

What hold Sara's experiences will continue to exercise on her imagination remains to be seen, and to be influenced by what is to come – whether she will discover the fate of her children, or the children themselves, and much besides. All this will be played out in social space, at present one in which as an asylum seeker she still carries little weight (as she knows only too well); one day she might well be back in Rwanda and with a different set of constraints and possibilities. The core dimension of most modern warfare is that it is total; it aims for the destruction of worlds (Summerfield, 1999b). This renders life incoherent. What Sara faces in the longer term may perhaps fairly be seen as a struggle to recover a sense of coherence, the absence of which is bad for anyone. But this is not a struggle apart: it is subsumed within, and represented by, the practical struggle to recover agency and to rebuild a life that endures, and even be worth enduring.

REFERENCES

African Rights (1995) *Rwanda not so Innocent. When Women Become Killers.* London: African Rights.
Argenti-Pillen, A. (2000) The discourse on trauma in non-Western cultural contexts: contributions of an ethnographic method. In Shalev, A., Yehuda, R. & McFarlane, A. (eds.), *International Handbook of Human Response to Trauma.* New York: Kluwer/Plenum, pp. 87-102.
Baluchi, B. (1999) *Beyond Urgent: Towards a Strategy for Mental Health.* London: Kimia Institute.
Boomstra, R. & Kramer, S. A. (1997) *Cultuurverschillen in interacties tussen hulpverleners en vluchtelingen.* Utrecht: ISOR.
Bracken, P. (1998) Hidden agendas: deconstructing post-traumatic stress disorder. In: Bracken, P. & Petty, C. (eds.), *Rethinking the Trauma of War.* New York: Free Association Books.
Bracken, P. (2000) Outside the magic circle: meaning and mental illness in the postmodern age. In: Centres for Disease Control Prevention, 1999, *A Mental Health Assessment in Kosovo.* International Emergency and Refugee Health Branch, CDC.
Dahoud, O. & Pelosi, A. (1989) The work of the Somali Counseling Program in the UK, *Bulletin of the Royal College of Psychiatrists 13,* 619-60.
De Jong, K., Mulhern, M., Ford, N., van der Kam, S. & Kleber, R. (2000) The trauma of war in Sierra Leone. *The Lancet 355,* 2067-2070.
Eastmond, M. (1998) Nationalist discourses and the construction of difference: Bosnian Muslim referees in Sweden. *Journal of Refugee Studies 11,* 161-181.
Foxen, P. (2000) Cacophony of voices: A K'iche' Mayan narrative of remembrance and forgetting, *Transcultural Psychiatry 37,* 355-381.
Gorst-Unsworth, C. & Goldenberg, E. (1998) Psychological sequelae of torture and organised violence suffered by refugees from Iraq. Trauma-related factors compared to social factors in exile. *British Journal of Psychiatry 172,* 90-94.
Hacking, I. (1996) *Rewriting the Soul. Multiple Personality and the Sciences of Memory.* Princeton: Princeton University Press.
Harrell Bond, B. (1999) The experience of refugees as recipients of aid. In A. Ager (ed.), *Refugees. Perspectives on the Experience of Forced Migration.* Gaskell: London, 136-168.
Ingleby, D. (1989) Critical psychology in relation to political repression and violence. *International Journal of Mental Health 17,* 16-28.
Kahn, R., Wise, P., Kennedy, B. & Kawachi, I. (2000) State income inequality, household income, and maternal mental and physical health: cross sectional national survey. *British Medical Journal 321,* 1311-1315.
Kaminer, D., Stein, D., Mbanga, I. & Zungu-Dirwayi, N. (2001) The Truth and Reconciliation Commission in South Africa: relation to psychiatric status and forgiveness among survivors of human rights abuses. *British Journal of Psychiatry 178,* 373-377.
Kawachi, I., Kennedy, B. (1997) Health and social cohesion: why care about income inequality? *British Medical Journal, 314,* 1037-1040.
Kenardy, J. (2000) The current status of psychological debriefing. *British Medical Journal 321,* 1032-1033.
Kirmayer, L. & Young, A. (1998) Culture and somatization: clinical, epidemiological and ethnographic perspectives. *Psychosomatic Medicine 60,* 420-429.
Kleinman, A. & Good, B. (eds.) (1985), *Culture and Depression: Studies in the Anthropology and Cross-Cultural Psychiatry of Affect and Disorder.* Berkeley: University of California Press.
Kleinman, A. (1987) Anthropology and psychiatry: The role of culture in cross-cultural research on illness, *British Journal of Psychiatry,* 151: 447-454.
Last, M. (2000) Healing the Social Wounds of War. *Medicine, Conflict and Survival 16,* 370-382.
Levi, P.1(988) *The Drowned and the Saved.* Harmondsworth: Penguin Books.

Lin, E., Carter, W. & Kleinman, A. (1985) An exploration of somatization among Asian refugees and immigrants in primary care. *American Journal of Public Health 75*, 1080-1084.

Littlewood, R. (1990) From categories to contexts: A decade of the 'new cross-cultural psychiatry'. *British Journal of Psychiatry* 156:308-327.

Marsella, A. & White, S. (eds.) (1982) *Cultural Conceptions of Mental Health and Therapy*. Dordrecht: Reidel.

Mayou, R., Ehlers, A. & Hobbs, M. (2000) Psychological debriefing for road traffic victims. Three-year follow-up of a randomised controlled trial. *British Journal of Psychiatry 176*, 589-593.

McAfee, B. (1998) *Instead of Medicine. Report of the Bosnian Mental Health Pilot Project*. London: Refugee Action.

Said, E. (1993) *Culture and Imperialism*. London: Chatto & Windus.

Skultans, V. (1998) *The Testimony of Lives: Narrative and Memory in Post-Soviet Latvia*. London: Routledge.

Smith, R. (1992) Without work all life goes rotten. *British Medical Journal 305*, 972.

Southwick, S., Morgan, C., Nicolaou A. & Charney, D. (1997) Consistency of memory for combat-related traumatic events in veterans of Operation Desert Storm. *American Journal of Psychiatry 154*, 173-177.

Steen, A. (1993) Refugee resettlement: Denmark and Britain compared. *Refugee Participation Newsletter 14*. Oxford: Refugee Studies Program.

Summerfield, D. (1997) South Africa: does a truth commission promote social reconciliation? *British Medical Journal 315*, 1393.

Summerfield, D. (1999a) A critique of seven assumptions behind psychological trauma programs in war-affected areas. *Social Science & Medicine 48*, 1449-1462.

Summerfield, D. (1999b) Sociocultural dimensions of war, conflict and displacement. In: *Refugees. Perspectives on the Experience of Forced Migration*. London: Gaskell, 111-135.

Summerfield, D. (2000) Childhood, War, Refugeedom and 'Trauma': Three Core Questions for Mental Health Professionals. *Transcultural Psychiatry 37*, 417-434.

Summerfield, D. (2001) The invention of post-traumatic stress disorder and the social usefulness of a psychiatric category. *British Medical Journal 322*, 95-98.

Taussig, M. (1980) Reification and the consciousness of the patient. *Social Science & Medicine 148*, 3-13.

Wessely, S., Rose, S. & Bisson, J. (1998) A systematic review of brief psychological interventions ('debriefing') for the treatment of immediate trauma related symptoms and the prevention of post traumatic stress disorder (Cochrane Review). *The Cochrane Library 2*. Oxford: Update Software.

Wilkinson, R. (1996) *Unhealthy Societies: the Afflictions of Inequality*. London: Routledge.

Young, A. (1995) *The Harmony of Illusions: Inventing Post-Traumatic Stress Disorder*. Princeton, NJ: Princeton University Press.

Zarowsky, C. (2000) Trauma Stories: Violence, Emotion and Politics in Somali Ethiopia. *Transcultural Psychiatry 37*, 383-402.

7. MENTAL HEALTH CARE FOR REFUGEE CHILDREN IN EXILE

Anders Hjern and Olle Jeppsson[1]

1. INTRODUCTION

The effects of warfare and political violence on the mental health of children have received increasing attention over the last few decades. In many recent armed conflicts the majority of the victims have not been soldiers, but women and children. Even when children and their caregivers succeed in finding refuge in another country, substantial psychosocial problems often remain as a result of pre-flight experiences and the difficulties of resettlement.

Scandinavian studies of the mental health of newly settled children in families from the Middle East and Latin America have yielded broadly comparable results; with 35 – 50% of children being judged as suffering from poor mental health (Almqqvist & Brandell-Forsberg, 1995; Hjern et al.. 1998; Ljungberg-Miklos, 1989; Montgomery, 1998; Svedin et al.. 1994). However, the psychosocial situation of the refugee child newly settled in exile is complex, and not all studies demonstrate such high rates of poor mental health. Studies of South-East Asian refugee children in Australia (Krupinski & Burrows, 1986) and Bosnian children in Sweden (Angel et al.., 2001) have indicated a general level of mental health which in some respects is actually better than that of the general child population in the country of reception.

Figure 1 presents an ecological model that identifies some of the major factors that should be taken into account in the provision of the mental health care of refugee children in exile (Bronfenbrenner 1986; Gibson 1989). The model distinguishes three levels of factors which can influence the well-being of children:

(1) stress experienced by the children themselves;
(2) available social support;
(3) the societal, political and cultural context.

---
[1] Olle Jeppsson Department of Pediatrics, Huddinge University Hospital, Karolinska Institutet, Stockholm, Sweden. Anders Hjern, National Board of Health and Welfare, Centre for Epidemiology, Stockholm, Sweden.

Figure 1. An ecological model of the psychosocial situation of refugee children in exile

Level 1: *STRESS*	• Organized Violence • Uprooting

Level 2: *SOCIAL SUPPORT*	• Family • Social Network

Level 3: *CONTEXT*	• Socio-economic situation in exile • Culture-specific discourse of childhood and mental health • Political situation in home country

Level One: Stress

All refugee children have experienced *forced migration*. They have been compelled to leave their home at short notice for reasons they may not understand. They are confronted with a new environment and with an unfamiliar culture and language. Several authors have described the child's reactions to these stressors as an 'immigrant crisis' (Aronowitz 1984; Eisenbruch 1988).

Many refugee children have been exposed to single or multiple incidents of political violence. For some children the threat of violence has been an important part of their environment for long periods of time, forcing adaptations of a more 'chronic' nature (Garbarino 1992).

Level Two: Social support

A large body of research (e.g. Caplan 1981) supports the importance of social support systems for maintaining mental health. Most refugee families in exile leave important parts, or perhaps all, of their social support system in their home country. This makes refugees particularly dependent on the support of their nuclear family and the refugee community in the host country. Migration and exposure to organized violence can affect family interaction in a negative way, with significant effects on the mental health of children (Agger and Jensen, 1989; Becker et al., 1987; Figley and McCubbin, 1983).

Level Three: Societal, cultural and political context

On a third level, the wider context of the psychosocial situation of refugees are considered, including obvious social variables such as employment, availability of schooling, day-care services and housing. The legal status of the refugee family, the attitudes of the population in resettlement countries and the culture-specific discourses of childhood and mental health are other important contextual factors that shape the matrix for the interactions of the child with his environment in exile.

Another important dimension in the context of refugee mental health is the political situation in the home country. Ongoing events in the home country and relationships with political movements at home and in exile are important elements in the formation of plans for the future and giving meaning to past events (Barudy 1989).

In the following pages we will present some experiences from our work with refugee children, focusing on different levels of this model. We will start with the traumatic stress approach, which has been very influential in Scandinavia. Then we will discuss an alternative approach based on social support and intervention on a societal level. Finally we will turn to the particular situation of refugee children that live illegally in exile, as an example of families for whom interventions on such a societal level are particularly important.

2. THE CONCEPT OF TRAUMATIC STRESS IN MENTAL HEALTH PROGRAMS FOR REFUGEE CHILDREN

American psychiatrists first used the term Post-Traumatic Stress Disorder (PTSD) in 1980 in order to describe the main elements of mental disturbances following psychic trauma (American Psychiatric Association, 1980). It subsequently gained widespread use in adult psychiatric clinical work with trauma victims and is currently a major topic in adult psychiatric research. Child psychiatrists too, have noted that the mental disturbances of children show many similarities to those of adults, and began to use the concept of PTSD in clinical practice and research in the latter part of the 1980´s (Eth & Pynoos 1985).

Epidemiological studies in Scandinavia have identified experiences of war and political persecution in the home country as important risk factors for mental health shortly after arrival in the resettlement country (Almqqvist & Brandell-Forsberg, 1995; Hjern et al., 1998; Ljungberg-Miklos, 1989; Montgomery, 1998; Svedin et al.., 1994). This has given the PTSD concept an important role in preventive efforts for refugee children in exile. The concept has also been introduced by Western relief agencies into health programs for children in war and disaster situations in Western countries such as ex-Yugoslavia (Kuterovac & Dyregrov, 1994), in non-Western contexts like the Middle East (Macksoud, 1992), and in war-stricken African countries such as Mozambique (Boothby et al., 1991) and Rwanda (Gupta, 1996). Group methods adapted to the situation of asylum seekers in exile have been developed and were used quite extensively in Sweden with refugee children from Bosnia in 1993-94 (Angel & Hjern, 2004).

The PTSD approach in mental health programs has been questioned from different angles. The next section demonstrates some aspects of the traumatic stress discourse that we have found problematic in our research and clinical work with refugee children in exile in Sweden and Kenya.

2.1. Trauma and the long-term adaptation of refugee children in exile

In a prospective study of refugee children from Chile and the Middle East in Stockholm, we had the opportunity to describe their mental health in relation to traumatic stress in the home country and time in exile. The study included 63 refugee children, 2–15 years of age when they first set foot on Swedish soil in 1986-87 (Hjern et al.. 1998; Hjern et al.. 2000). Two-thirds of the children had personally experienced political violence during war and/or persecution in the home country. High levels of poor mental health were recorded during the children's first 18 months in Sweden; 46% of the children were rated as having poor mental health after 5 months and 44 % after 18 months in Sweden.

In 1993-94, 49 of these children were investigated again in parent, teacher and child interviews. The rate of poor mental health had fallen significantly to 24% in parent interviews and 18% in teacher interviews. Only one neurologically damaged child fulfilled the criteria of PTSD, and only another three children reported symptoms that indicated they might be re-experiencing or trying to avoid remembering traumatic events. Other symptoms related to PTSD such as fears, anxiety, sleep disturbances and being easily startled were common during the first 18 months in Sweden, but were rare in the follow-up study, six to seven years after settlement in Sweden. Instead, the most worrying signs among the refugee children in this follow-up research were many incidents of low moods and loneliness (Hjern et al., 2000).

In 1994 Angel et al. (2001) used the same methods to describe the mental health situation of 99 school-aged refugee children from Bosnia 12-24 months after resettlement in Växjö, Sweden. The general level of poor mental health was surprisingly low: no more than 11% were described as having poor mental health, despite fairly high levels of sleeping disturbances, separation anxiety and depressed mood. Children from the area of Prijedor in northern Bosnia, who had experienced very severe 'ethnic cleansing' which often included experiences in the concentration camps of Omarska and Trnoplje, were more often reported to be in distress with symptoms of PTSD as well as depression and anxiety. Four years later (Angel et al., 2004) 11 of the Prijedor children were interviewed again and compared with age- and sex-matched controls from the rest of the study population. Most of them (8) still had symptoms of re-experiencing and/or avoidance of memories of these events, but only one fulfilled the full criteria of the PTSD-syndrome. Apart from the specific PTSD symptoms, however, these children showed few signs of child psychiatric disturbances, either in their own reports or in the reports of their parents. In the first study in 1994 the children from Prijedor had significantly higher scores of poor mental health than the comparison group, but these differences had disappeared in the follow-up.

These studies – supported by many others – demonstrated that certain symptoms related to the PTSD concept are common among refugee children during the first years in exile. It seems difficult however, to a make a clear distinction between cases with PTSD and children with no post-traumatic suffering. The situation is better described as a continuum of children who have similar symptoms of varying intensity. Five to seven years after settlement in Sweden, child psychiatric symptoms seem to be much less common despite few psychotherapeutic interventions, therefore suggesting that most children have the capability to recover from these symptoms without professional help. Specific symptoms related to distressful memories may remain but rarely seem to interfere with the activities of daily life. Studies in adulthood of children exposed to Nazi persecution (Keilsson 1992; Moskovitz 1985), the Greek Civil war in 1948-9 (Dalianis-Karambatzikis, 1994) and Kampuchea (Kinzie et al., 1989) have demonstrated a similar capability of children to recover from, or at least live with, symptoms of traumatic stress.

2.2. Transcultural aspects of the trauma concept in childhood

2.2.1. Childhood as a social construction

In meeting recently settled families from non-Western cultural backgrounds, we are reminded of the importance of the cultural context in which child health is promoted in Europe. In a professional Western model, children are seen as different from adults due to a set of biological and psychological – as opposed to social – characteristics. Children also tend to be seen as vulnerable and are attributed with special disabilities that make their protection and nurture a matter of great importance. Various periods and phases of childhood are considered to be universal and made up by recognizable developmental stages. For optimal development and health, a favorable set of personal, environmental and family conditions are required. Most of what is done in preventive programs has, in one way or another, to do with promoting these favorable conditions.

It is easy to forget that this social construction of childhood is historically and culturally tied to the social and economic conditions of Europe and North America in the last century (Boyden, 1994). Most refugee parents have some experience of the social construction of childhood in Western countries from their home country – it is, after all, the dominant framework among well educated people in the world today – but they may nevertheless feel alien to many aspects of Western child health programs. Not all parents in all refugee communities necessarily share the view that children are particularly vulnerable to situations of stress, which is an important assumption in most mental health programs for refugee children in Europe. The example of unaccompanied minors in Sudan, as described in Chapter 4 of this book, demonstrates that the cultural context of childhood may have very significant implications for the way in which traumatic stress is perceived and expressed. Awareness of this culture-dependence is an important starting point for mental health programs for refugee children.

2.3. Attitudes towards discussing past suffering

The basic assumption underlining most PTSD-centered mental health care is that child victims of war cannot recover properly without emotionally ventilating, or 'working through' their war experiences (Summerfield 1999). In mental health programs with this perspective, working through is facilitated by offering children the possibility of express-ing their experiences in drawings, drama, group discussions and so on. This principle is familiar to most members of societies with a strong Christian influence, where the impor-tance of confession and sharing distress has been preached in Christian communities since 200-300 AD (Pennebaker, 1997). Though quite a few non-Western cultures have similar beliefs, many others discourage disclosure (Wellenkamp, 1997). Mozambicans, for example, talk about forgetting as their normative means of coping. Ethiopians call this 'active forgetting' (Summerfield, 1999).

In a study of Bosnian school children shortly after their arrival in Sweden, parents were asked about how they handled the traumatic events in the family (Angel et al.,

2001). Sixty-nine percent of parents said that they actively tried not to talk with their children about the war. The most common reason given for this was that they thought that their children were better off not being reminded of their suffering in the home country. When the data was analyzed for the effects of parental attitudes towards discussing the war, it was found that for children who had experienced many war stresses, talking about these experiences seemed not to ameliorate but to exacerbate their negative effects. This contrasts greatly with the positive effects of sharing distress found among British school-children who survived a ferry disaster (Yule, 1992). These divergent effects of working through seem to indicate that the effect of a working-through program in one context cannot automatically be translated to a different population with a different cultural discourse for dealing with painful memories.

2.4. Screening for Traumatic Stress

Mental health professionals who cross over to public health care tend to be strong advocates of screening in child health care programs. European child health care programs rely heavily on screening for problems such neuro-psychiatric deficiencies, language problems and mental retardation. A number of other screening programs have been implemented on a small scale, such as screening for autism in babies and depression in mothers of young children. What makes screening such a natural public health activity for clinicians is its similarity to clinical work, in that it is individually oriented and usually leads to a treatment for which a clinician is needed. Therefore it is not surprising that many mental health professionals in Europe advocate the screening of refugee children for PTSD, so that suffering children and families can be offered an appropriate individual treatment.

Screening is a very common method in child health care in the Western world, and over the years much experience has been gained about when and how to use it. Criteria for those health problems that may require screening have been defined as follows (Hall, 1996):

- The problem should have a documented long lasting effect on the health or life quality of the individual;
- There must be methods that can effectively separate potential patients from healthy individuals;
- There is a treatment which has been rigorously evaluated and proven to be effective.
- There are enough resources to treat all identified potential cases.

In the light of the studies mentioned above, it is difficult to see that PTSD fulfills these criteria. Even the criterion for an evidence-based treatment for PTSD in childhood has been questioned in some reviews (e.g. Pfefferbaum, 1997). If we add the ethical dilemma of screening for a health problem in a refugee population that is often unfamiliar with the concept of traumatization and actively opposes working-through therapy, it must be concluded that there are few contexts where screening for PTSD is good practice.

3. AN APPROACH BASED ON SOCIAL SUPPORT AND INTERVENTION ON A SOCIETAL LEVEL

The fact that the discourse of traumatic stress in prevention of mental health problems of refugee children in exile has important shortcomings should not discourage us. Refugee children are in a vulnerable position in their host societies. Health professionals can make important contributions to prevent that vulnerability developing into mental health problems. There are alternatives to the trauma approach. In what follows we will give examples of approaches that can be used in the creation of preventive mental health programs for refugee children.

3.1. Social network

The social network provides social support; this can include a mother and a father, grandparents, aunts and uncles and cousins, friends and their relatives, schoolteachers and day-care personnel, neighbors, social workers, nurses and doctors and so on. There are people you know and who know you, and who know each other. There is a language and a landscape you are acquainted with that helps you create a somewhat predictable world. Many channels and persons provide for a child's need for support, joy, play, consolation, education, governance, food for growth, self-respect and development. These people support each other: when one fails there is often another one to help; what one cannot give, another can. In everyday life you tend not even to think about it.

The refugee child has to leave this well-known world. For reasons that are not always clear to him, the family settles in a new country. Most of the network is gone. In exile, the refugee family is left on its own to recreate a functioning social support system. This is no easy task in a new country with an unfamiliar culture and language. Facilitating the recreative process and finding a constructive role for the health professional in this new social support system are important aspects of mental health care programs for refugees.

3.2. The refugee community

The refugee community is important for the well-being of refugees (Angel et al., 2001; Stubbs & Sorya, 1996; Richman, 1998). On the one hand, being part of a community helps to maintain a valid political and religious meaning system, which is crucial for political refugees. The community also offers a social matrix in which the lost social network can be reconstituted, and experiences of loss and persecution expressed and shared. On the other hand, some communities crumble under the heavy load of life in exile and create destructive social patterns where powerlessness, poverty and frustration create hostility towards newcomers. Assisting in the creation of strong communities is a key area in prevention of mental health problems in refugees.

Social work methods for community work and community development have been developed in deprived areas in big cities in Europe. These methods have also been found to be appropriate for social work with refugee communities (Stubbs & Soraya, 1996). Political refugees are by definition often quite experienced organizers and used to expressing themselves politically, which may be why this approach is often so well accepted by refugee populations. Community projects often have a broad approach in which refugees set the agenda themselves. The focus is often on practical aspects of life such as housing, education and employment. From a psychosocial point of view it seems evident that these projects help to create a more healthy social environment where frustration can be channeled into constructive political terms, while simultaneously creating a sense of autonomy and self-respect.

Health professionals from the refugee population can be an important nucleus for community projects with a focus on health. There are good examples of this kind from the Latin American community in Belgium as well as from the Bosnian community in Sweden. In a similar way, community projects may focus on the needs of the children in the refugee community. Thus, a Latin American collective in Leuven (Belgium) developed ways of supporting Latin American children in exile by creating *talleres* (workshops) in the early 1980's (COLAT, 1982). In the *talleres* children met once a week in different kinds of creative activities that include learning songs and dances from their home country. During the summer the groups go to camp together with a similar curriculum. Many refugee communities use similar kinds of child groups to create social support within the framework of religious, political or sports organizations.

3.3. Supportive environments

Children in most northern European societies spend a considerable part of their childhood in institutions like day care, schools, and after-school homes. How newly settled refugee children are cared for within these institutions should be of major concern for preventive mental health programs. In many Swedish schools there are introduction classes where newly settled children are taken care of in small groups until the children know the language well enough to be integrated into normal classes. From a psychosocial viewpoint these introduction classes can be seen as supportive environments where a caring adult gives the children individual attention and support. Teachers in smaller introduction classes also have much more opportunity for parent collaboration and support.

Day care centers for full day or half day care for pre-school children is another key arena for newly settled refugee children. Many parents and children need considerable time to get acquainted with this kind of group care, which is quite often a completely new experience for them. But for children in the transitional situation of the newly settled refugee child, a well-functioning day care center can be an extremely important island of stable social relations and play.

3.4. Host families

Sometimes refugee families settle in areas where there are few compatriots. These families are easily isolated and may need help to break this isolation. Awarding each refugee family a host family in the receiving community is one way of facilitating the creation of a social network. The host family can also serve as a useful informal guide into the new society.

3.5. The role of the health professional

Child health professionals, such as nurses in schools and child health centers have an important role in the social support system of the newly settled refugee family. They offer the possibility for children to meet other children in different activities, and can provide information for parents such as where to go when children are ill or in need of psychiatric counseling. In individual or group conversations they can provide social support and an important platform for discussion about how to cope with being a parent in a new society with an unfamiliar culture.

3.6. Intervention on a societal level

There are few children in Europe today whose living conditions are as much defined by specific regulations and policies as those of refugee children. Immigrant and refugee policy is usually made with adult refugees in mind, and the fact that some 25-30% of the populations are children is usually forgotten. Child health professionals have an important task in getting involved in the process of legislation as well as the creation of refugee reception programs in the local community that respect the need for adequate health services, structured activities for pre-school children and good quality education for the older children.

4. A PROGRAM FOR REFUGEE CHILD HEALTH IN STOCKHOLM

When the authors of this article were given the responsibility of developing a public health strategy for the reception of refugee children in the greater Stockholm area, an approach based on social support and societal intervention was preferred to a trauma-centered approach. In this strategy, all newly settled refugee children are considered to be in a position of vulnerability, and interventions target all children in the refugee population (see Table 1).

4.1. Introduction and information

Existing child and school health institutions were given the task of introducing the newly settled refugee families and their children to the health system in Stockholm. Basic child health programs like vaccination, injury prevention, dental health and basic medical screening were updated. Screening for certain infectious disorders like hepatitis B and tuberculosis was arranged in collaboration with local health centers.

Information was given about the possibilities of group activities for the children, and nurses were encouraged to assist parents in getting children enrolled in the available services. Information about the nature and availability of child psychiatric care in Sweden was given in the context of general questions about the health of the children. No screening for mental health problems took place, but when parents or children themselves expressed a wish to get in touch with child psychiatric services, they were helped to do so.

A poor system of information regarding the whereabouts of asylum-seeker children in their journey from the national immigration services to primary care was identified as a major obstacle for asylum-seeker children to get in touch with child health centers. This system was improved by establishing a direct link between child health services and immigration services, which meant that most asylum-seeker children could be, offered a child health center appointment within a few weeks of settling in Stockholm.

Table 1. A population-based mental health program for refugee children in exile

---

1. Introduction and information
(schools, child health care centers, government agencies etc):
- information (including possibilities for psychiatric and child psychiatric treatment)
- update of basic child health programs.

2 .Parent support
- individual support through child health nurses
- parent groups

3. Supportive environments
- introduction classes in schools (to provide individualized support and teaching during the first months/year in the new country)
- nursery school programs
- network facilitation: aid to create organizations, contact families

4.Basic child health and medical care for 'illegal' children
- child health center for 'illegals'
- network of health professionals

5.Secondary care
- 'Experts' educate and guide the first-line investigators and/or treat patients who are put forward by their parents or in their daily environment (school, day care)
- advocacy

4.2. Parent support

Nurses in child health centers were encouraged to establish a continuing dialogue with refugee parents. Visits for vaccinations and other basic child health care activities form a good framework for discussing themes related to parenthood and child health in the Swedish society. To this end parent groups were organized in areas where refugee families were clustered in transitional housing.

4.3. Supportive environments

In the greater Stockholm area, a lack of group activities for asylum-seeker children of pre-school age and the lack of introduction classes in certain communities were identified as the major weaknesses in the school system for newly settled refugee children. Advocacy for such possibilities was an important part of the mental health program and was quite successful for the pre-schoolers.

4.4. Secondary care

The mental health program for refugee children in Stockholm was based around a small nucleus of professionals with a particular interest in the situation of refugee children. This group tried to develop appropriate methods that could be used in primary care settings, such as a structured introduction program for refugee children in child health and school health centers, and parent groups. Information about the psychosocial situation of refugees and working methods was documented in pamphlets that were distributed to the primary care centers in Stockholm and used in a series of seminars for primary care givers. The group also provided advice for primary care professionals by telephone and undertook frequent visits to key centers in areas with many refugees.

In certain areas with many refugees, the group worked closely with schools and day care centers, providing support to teachers and performing individual investigations of children with who had been identified as having particular learning and emotional problems.

A very important task for the expert group was advocacy. This advocacy operated on a local level, in trying to improve the school and day care situation through identifying weaknesses and suggesting alternatives, and on a political level, where advocacy for the rights of 'undocumented' children for medical care and education was the most important demand on the agenda.

5. MENTAL HEALTH CARE FOR 'UNDOCUMENTED CHILDREN'

Refugee children who reside illegally ('undocumented') in Europe stand out as a group where action on a societal level is particularly urgent. In northern Europe, this group of children is made up mainly of children in refugee families whose application for asylum has been turned down. In southern Europe, these children can be counted in hundreds of thousands, a considerable proportion being refugees from war and persecution in the Balkans, Africa and the Middle East (Hjern & Bouvier, 2004).

Many European societies today grant certain basic rights for medical and health care and education to children who are residing illegally in their society. Spain and Italy are examples of societies where ways have been found to accommodate this group of children inside the public health and medical care system as well as in the public school system. Sweden recently created possibilities for state-funded health and medical care for these children but left out rights to education.

The life of 'undocumented children' is defined by their lack of basic rights of housing, of education, of food and proper clothing. They move from place to place; their houses never become homes. Children have to stay indoors, keep silent and not attract attention. They do not have enough money. They lose the friends they had, and in losing their school or day-care, they lose acquired knowledge. All the needs formerly provided by many persons and channels now have to be provided by the parents who are sad, afraid and poor.

The 'undocumented child' has almost never asked to become a refugee, and has had few, if any, possibilities to influence either the situation in his homeland or the decision to flee and hide. He is obviously a suffering, unprotected, innocent third party in the conflict going on between his parents and the State. Humanity demands the creation of special rules and laws of protection for these children.

Strange as it may sound, the very efficiency and logical consistency of the modern State may make the situation of these children even more difficult. If for example there is a decision to expel the family, there is no exception, no special rule for the child. If he is not wanted by the State he cannot expect to be wanted by any of its official ramifications, be it the police, education or the medical sector. Former societies were less efficient, less logically congruent and strangely enough more human. There were no resources to track down people wherever they may be: not all civil servants behaved exactly alike. There was a space for practical reasoning, exceptions, illogical decisions and mercy. For – as Dostoyevski put it – 'You have only facts, no affection, thus it becomes wrong'.

In pre-modern societies, rules based on morality were not necessarily rules of the State and sprang from goodwill, not from logic. You could not chase and kill an enemy inside a church, but laid down your weapons before entering. You could not rob and kill a foreign traveler in alien lands: instead, you had to provide food and shelter. Safe havens were created as the result of individuals' own experiences and sense of vulnerability on the roads in unfamiliar surroundings.

Such safe havens should be provided for the 'undocumented child'. He should be able to go to school or to Kindergarten and to attend medical care without fear. He should never be regarded as a possible hostage to enable the seizure of his parents. Either the State must be less efficient in these matters, or better still; it should take a decision to provide the child with such safety.

Finally, these problems are, as Henri Dunant (founder of the International Red Cross) realized, also problems for the professionals taking care of the children. Health professionals should care for clients regardless of social, religious or legal status. The medical professional oath solemnly states that, "The doctor should let himself be led by the commandments of humanitarianism and honor, and the health of his patient should be his primary goal". The 'undocumented' child tests the humanitarian standards of the professional as well as of the State. If we cannot stand the test today when it actually costs us so little, how will it be in hard times? When those unwanted by the State seek our help, must we stand up for the opinions of this State? Does everyone always have to obey? What happens then with health professionals? Do we break the trust of our patients? It is obvious that child health professionals have a duty not only to provide care for individual 'illegal' children, but also act on the policy level. Those politicians responsible should not be allowed to forget that these children exist, that they need better health and medical care than any other children in our society because of their very harsh living conditions, and that the UN Convention of the Child grants them these rights.

REFERENCES

Agger, I., and Jensen, S. B. (1989) Coupes in Exile: political consciousness as an element in the psychosexual dynamics of a Latin American refugee couple. *Sexual and marital therapy 4*, 101-108.

Almqvist K, Brandell-Forsberg M. (1995) Iranian refugee children in Sweden: effects of organized violence and forced migration on preschool children. *American Journal of Orthopsychiatry 65*, 225-237.

Almqvist K, Brandell M. (1997) Refugee children in Sweden: post-traumatic stress disorder in Iranian preschool children exposed to organized violence. *Child Abuse & Neglect 4*, 351-366.

Angel, B., Hjern, A. & Ingleby, D. (2001) Effects of war and organized violence on children: a study of Bosnian refugees in Sweden. *American Journal of Orthopsychiatry 71*, 4-15.

Angel B., Almqvist, K., Ingleby, D. & Hjern, A. (2004). Effects of war and organized violence on children: a 4-year follow-up study of Bosnians in Växjö. Unpublished report.

Angel, B., and Hjern, A. (2004) *Att möta flyktingbarn*. Lund: Studentlitteratur.

Aronowitz, M. (1984) The social and emotional adjustment of immigrant children. *International Migration Review 18*, 237-257.

Barudy, J. (1989) A programme of mental health for political refugees: Dealing with the invisible pain of political exile. *Social Science & Medicine 28*, 715-727.

Becker, D., Maggi, A., and Domínguez, R. (1987) *Tortura y dano familiar, Trauma, duelo y reparación – Una experiencia de trabajo psicosocial en Chile*. Madrid: Editorial Interamericana.

Brandell-Forsberg, M., and Almqvist, K. (1997) *"Bildverkstaden" – Projektet för traumatiserade flyktingbarn – Undersökning och behandling av barn i förberedelseklasser*. Karlstad: Tryckarna Text & Reklam AB.

Bronfenbrenner, U. (1986) Ecology of the family as a context for human development: Research perspectives. *Developmental Psychology 22*, 723-742..

Caplan, G. (1981) Mastery of stress: psychosocial aspects. *American Journal of Psychiatry 138*, 413-20.

COLAT (1982) Psicopatologia de la tortura y el Exilio. Madrid: Editiorial Fundamentos.

Dalianis-Karambatzakis, A. M. (1994) *Children in turmoil during the Greek civil war 1946-49: today's adults. A longitudinal study on children confined with their mothers in prison*. Stockholm: Karolinska Institutet.

Eisenbruch, M. (1988) The mental health of refugee children and their cultural development. *International Migration Review 22*, 282-300.

Eth., S. & Pynoos. R. (eds.) (1985) *Post-traumatic stress disorder in children*. Washington DC.: American Psychiatric Press. ·

Figley, C. R. & McCubbin, H. I. (1983) *Stress and the Family : Volume II : Coping with Catastrophe*, Vol. II. New York: Brunner/Mazel.

Garbarino, J. (1992) Developmental consequences of living in dangerous and unstable environment: the situation of refugee children. In McCallin, M. (ed.), T*he psychological well-being of refugee children. Research, practice and policy issues*. Geneva: International Child Bureau.

Gibson, K. (1989) Children in political violence. *Social Science & Medicine 28*, 659-667.

Hall, D.M.B. (1996) *Health for all children*. Third Edition. Oxford: Oxford University Press.

Hjern, A., Angel, B. & Jeppson, O. (1998) Political violence, family stress and mental health of refugee children in exile. *Scandinavian Journal of Social Medicine 26*,18-25.

Hjern, A., Angel, B.& Jeppson, O. (2000) Organised violence and mental health in refugee children – A six year follow-up. *Acta Paediatrica 89*, 722-727.

Hjern, A. & Bouvier, F. (2004). Migrant children – a challenge for paediatricians. *Acta Paediatrica*, in press.

Keilson, H. (1992) *Sequential traumatisation*. Jerusalem: Magnes Press.

Kinzie J.D., Sack., W., Angell, R., Clarke, G., Ben, R. (1989) A three-year follow-up of Cambodian young people traumatized as children. *Journal of the American Academy of Child & Adolescent Psychiatry 28*, 501–4.

Krupinski J., & Burrows, G. (1986*)* Psychiatric disorders in adolescents and young adults. In J. Krupinski (ed.), *The price of freedom*, 123-135. Sydney: Pergamon Press.

Ljungberg-Miklos, J. (1989) The mental health of refugee children [In Swedish]. *Socialmedicinsk Tidskrift 66*, 18-24.

Montgomery, E. (1998) Refugee children from the Middle East. *Scandinavian Journal of Social Medicine* (Suppl. 54).

Moskovitz, S. (1985) Longitudinal follow-up of child survivors of the holocaust. *Journal of the American Academy of Adolescent and Child Psychiatry 24*, 401-407.

Pennebaker, J.W. (ed.) (1997) *Opening up: The healing power of expressing emotions*. New York: Guilford Press.

Pfefferbaum, B. (1997) Posttraumatic stress disorder in children: A review of the past 10 years. *Journal of the American Academy of Adolescent and Child Psychiatry 36*,1503-1511.

Richman, N. (1998) Looking before and after: Refugees and asylum seekers in the west. In: Bracken, P.J. & Petty, C. (eds.), *Rethinking the trauma of war*. London: Free Association Books.

Stubbs, P. & Soroya, B.(1996) War trauma, psychosocial projects and social development in Croatia. *Medicine, Conflict and Survival 12*, 303-14.

Summerfield, D. (1999) A critique of seven assumptions behind psychological trauma programmes in war affected areas. *Social Science & Medicine 48*, 1449-62

Terr, L. C. (1991) Childhood traumas: an outline and overview. *American Journal of Psychiatry 148*,10-20.

Vogel, J.M. & Vernberg, E.M. (1993) Task force report. Part 1: Children's psychological responses to disasters. *Journal of Clinical Child Psychology 22*, 464-84.

Wellenkamp, J. (1997). Cultural similarities and differences regarding emotional disclosure: some examples from Indonesia and the Pacific. In: J. Pennebaker (ed.), *Opening up – The healing power of expressing emotions*, 293-311). New York: Guilford Press .

8. GETTING CLOSER
Methods of research with refugees and asylum seekers

Sander Kramer[1]

Not so long ago, the fundamental attitude in Western health care could be described as *paternalistic*. The doctor knew what was good for you; your task was to be grateful and carry out instructions. It was not important for you to understand the nature of your problem or the rationale behind the treatment. You were, literally, a *patient:* one to whom something is done.

Over the last few decades, however, an important shift has taken place in Western ideals of service delivery. In mental health, the 'patient' has become a 'client': active participation is seen as a precondition of successful treatment, and this entails that clients have to understand the thinking behind the treatment. In general health care – as in all service professions – increasing attention is paid to the 'matching' of supply and demand.

'Matching' has, in the first place, a *quantitative* meaning: people should be given what they need, not just what the service provider wants to give them. Just because your hospital is rather good at hip replacement operations does not mean that everybody should have them. Clients should be representative of the local population, taking certain risk factors into account. However, matching also concerns *qualitative* aspects of care delivery: client and professional should be on the same wavelength, the care given should be relevant and meaningful to the client. At first, service providers tried to improve this kind of matching by trying the change the views of the client (for example, through 'psycho-education'). Gradually, however, it became clear that professionals and service providers would also have to do their share of adapting, by taking more account of the needs of users and their ways of understanding their problems.

One way of realizing this goal of 'demand-driven' care is by encouraging feedback from users and inviting them to participate in the planning of services. In the Netherlands, for example, it has become almost obligatory for mental health services to set up a panel of (ex-)clients and their families, to provide advice on all kinds of organizational and sometimes even therapeutic matters. The disadvantage of this procedure is that it is hard to be sure that the people who find their way on to these panels are representative of those who use the services.

---

[1] Utrecht School of Governance, Utrecht University, The Netherlands.

Research on users' needs and their satisfaction with the services provided is another important tool for improving the match between supply and demand. In general, however, there are difficulties with research on (ex-)clients. Three types of problems can be distinguished:

1. *Methodological problems.* Making quantitative generalizations about people's needs and opinions is only possible if one uses standardized methods of data collection – but these methods may only succeed in picking up the phenomena which the researcher expects to find. Standardized questionnaires, check-lists and diagnostic instruments may fail to tap into the experiential world of users.

2. *Sampling problems.* How do we reach users, and what biases are involved in the way in which we select our research sample? If we confine ourselves to client populations, we will only obtain information about the people who find their way to the services. There are likely to be major differences between such people and others in need of care who do not seek or obtain help.

3. *Response biases.* How should we make allowance for clients' feelings of loyalty towards their caregiver, or the fact that their answers might reflect needs the clients hope their therapist will still fulfill? What difference does the *timing* of the questions make (for instance, should we ask about satisfaction just after a therapeutic encounter, or 6 months after the last visit?) Can we take for granted that respondents will be willing to confide in us, or understand how to answer our questions?

This chapter deals with the question of how it is possible to get closer to the perspective of service users – in particular, asylum seekers and refugees. The series of four studies which I will describe was carried out at Utrecht University from 1996 onwards. The first study was carried out in collaboration with Rinske Boomstra and was supervised by David Ingleby and Arie de Ruijter. The second and third studies were carried out by myself and the last study was carried out jointly with Julia Bala, Rob van Dijk and Ferko Öry.

The underlying aim of all these studies was to get closer to the perspective of asylum seekers and refugees themselves. I became interested in pursuing this line of research when I noticed, both in my professional work as a social worker and my study of the research literature, that very little attention was ever paid to what these groups themselves actually thought: what sorts of help they felt they needed, what they felt about the help they got.

In what follows I will present each of these studies in the same way, giving a short summary of the aims and methods of the project, presenting the results, discussing methodological pitfalls, and suggesting what conclusions can be drawn from each study for the improvement of services for asylum seekers and refugees.

1. CULTURAL DIFFERENCES IN INTERACTIONS BETWEEN REFUGEES AND SERVICE PROVIDERS

1.1. Aim and method

Aim. This first study (Boomstra and Kramer, 1997) was designed to explore the misunderstandings which may arise between mental health workers, social workers and other professionals and refugees as a result of cultural differences. Although several authors who have worked with refugees have claimed that cultural differences do not form a serious barrier to therapy with this group (see e.g. Van der Veer, 1992/1998), this conclusion seemed to us questionable in the light of the numerous problems that cultural differences are reported as posing in the mental health care of other migrants. Besides, the essence of such problems is that people are not aware that they exist; if misunderstandings are obvious, they can be cleared up, but if they are not, neither party may realize that anything is wrong. This was clearly illustrated in this study, where the participants seldom reported difficulties due to cultural barriers, though the findings revealed many misunderstandings.

Our interest was thus in the *interactions* between therapists and refugees. However, direct observation of therapy sessions was not deemed practical, so we collected information about the perceptions and opinions of each party. This approach had the advantage of uncovering many discrepancies and misunderstandings which would not have been evident simply from observing the interaction. Ideally, one should combine direct observation with the participants' own perceptions.

Sample. Eighteen therapists working with refugees were recruited from service providers in six sectors. These were community mental health centers, a specialized in-patient department serving refugees, a refugee health organization, local refugee council groups, social services and public health services. Recruitment of the professionals was on the basis of known interest in refugee problems and willingness to participate. This is unquestionably a biased selection, in that those recruited were particularly knowledgeable about the problems of refugees and particularly committed to their care. Our justification for this selectivity was that if problems are found in this group, they will almost certainly be found elsewhere.

In each sector, at least two therapists were approached. Each therapist had to chose one refugee from his or her practice as an example of a 'good' interaction and a second refugee as a 'difficult' or 'unsuccessful' interaction. In total, we were able to conduct and analyze interviews with 25 clients. This selection, too, is biased: it excludes clients who have dropped out of therapy. Again, however, we can assume that if there are problems among this group, there will be even more among the others. It is also important to remember that the sample may not be representative of people who never sought or were given therapy.

To conclude the study, a one-day workshop was held in which the researchers presented their findings to many of the participants in the study. Many insights which came up in this discussion were utilized when writing up the results. In this way, the workshop proved to be an extremely valuable source of additional data.

Theoretical framework The central concern of the research was the construction of meanings by refugees and therapists – in particular, meanings concerning psychic problems and their treatment, and the influence of cultural differences on these. In order to structure and analyze the interviews, models were used from two theoretical approaches in anthropology and communication studies.

1. Culture-bound views of illness and treatment were elucidated using Kleinman's (1981) concept of 'explanatory models'. This notion includes the illness concepts themselves, beliefs about the origins of illness, the form it takes, its progress and appropriate forms of treatment. Special attention was paid to the distinction between *internalizing* and *externalizing* medical systems (Young, 1979; Richters, 1996). Western medicine (including health care) typically emphasizes processes within the individual, while other approaches may have a more social and collective focus. Refugees in particular may include *political* dimensions of their problems in a way that Western therapists are not accustomed to doing.

2. The concept of 'meta-contract' (Rommetveit, 1974) was used to describe the structure of expectations about the therapeutic interaction. The 'meta-contract' comprises implicit assumptions about the purpose of an interaction, the role of the parties involved and the rules and conventions governing interaction.
    We assumed that explanatory models would be important determinants of the meta-contracts governing therapy, for such models incorporate notions about the 'sick role', the nature of the doctor/patient or therapist/client relationship (including the characteristics of a 'good patient' or 'good client'), and the goal and content of therapy.

The fundamental assumption of this study was that therapists and clients approach the interaction from culturally determined systems of interpretation, which may diverge substantially without the parties being aware of this. In successful interactions, agreement about the meta-contract which is to govern the relationship is reached through 'management of meanings'. When parties are unaware of the discrepancies between their meta-contracts, this cannot take place. Therapy is less likely to succeed when the parties do not realize that their interpretations diverge, or when they are unable to reconcile their differing interpretations.

If we attempt to characterize modern Western therapy forms in terms of explanatory models and meta-contracts, the most striking element is their 'democratic' nature. Like social relations in most other areas of life (see De Swaan, 1982), they are increasingly based on reciprocity and equality of status. The emphasis is on *negotiation*, the therapist being above all a *partner* and not an authoritarian expert. According to De Swaan, a 'good client' is articulate and prepared to look at problems objectivity and assume responsibility for them. The client accepts the constraints of the therapy and both parties keep its content to themselves. Whereas in traditional medicine (and even today in some branches of physical medicine) doctors essentially informed patients what was wrong with them and what they had to do about it, in modern practice the patient has something to say about both issues. Instead of the doctor being 'proactive' and the patient 'reactive', the roles are more equal.

The 'meta-contract' underlying most modern Western forms of therapy is firmly based on middle-class norms of self-expression, individualism, fostering autonomy, and tolerance. The more a client has been 'proto-professionalized' (i.e. educated in professional notions), the more he or she will share the meta-contract and explanatory model of the therapist. Conversely, some clients (particularly those who are not Western and/or middle-class) will come to therapy assuming a more directive, authoritarian model, with the therapist in the commanding role. For many migrants (according to Broekx et al., 1980) it is especially important to have clear confirmation of their sickness, because this justifies their inability to meet social responsibilities. Delving into strong emotions with strict professional detachment is also likely to strike those unacquainted with the conventions of therapy as artificial and unnatural – perhaps even as distant, indifferent or patronizing.

From the above it will be apparent that we came to the research with a fairly definite idea of where we could expect to find discrepancies. However, what is presented above as the theoretical framework was by no means completely in place at the beginning of the research. Only as data collection proceeded did it become clear where the emphases could most usefully be placed.

Data collection and analysis. Extended interviews were held with the 18 therapists and 25 clients in order to inventorize the views which both parties held about key issues and to compare the impressions they had of each other and of the therapeutic interaction. The key issues concerned the problems the client had and the nature of the help given. The interview was divided into distinct sections, dealing with:

- the admission process
- difficulties and complaints
- formulation of the 'problem' by client and therapist
- diagnosis
- choice of treatment and the way this was carried out
- general views on therapy for refugees.

In each section, the questions concerned not only the present case but also 'refugees in general'. Both therapist and client were asked about the extent to which they thought the case was representative of other refugees.

Operationalization of theoretical concepts. Questions about 'explanatory models' concerned the clients' difficulties and complaints (including the current living situation), the factors seen as causing his or her problem, the precise nature of the problem and the appropriate way of dealing with them. The same questions were given to both therapist and client. In order not to activate anxiety and distress we avoided questioning clients about traumatic experiences, though these were often spontaneously mentioned in relation to the treatment.

Opinions about the causes of problems were categorized in two ways: first, according to whether the factor mentioned was *social* or *individual* in nature, and second, whether it was *open to change* or *fixed*. In the analyses we tried to discover if the degree of consensus between therapist and client about the causes, nature and treatment of the problem was related to the success of the interaction.

Analysis of the data Interviews were tape-recorded, except in a few cases where this was objected to. The language was Dutch or English; sometimes an interpreter was used. The interviews were transcribed completely. A summary was made of each interview.

In formulating questions about the 'meta-contract', we were guided by Rommetveit's (1974) distinction between three aspects of the interaction which the 'meta-contract' covers: *mutual roles, assumed knowledge* and *motives.*

1. The first issue relating to the *mutual roles* of therapist and client was the question of how *symmetrical* the participants assume the interaction was supposed to be. If the therapist claimed to work in a 'client-centered' way, was this actually the case in the way topics of conversation or treatment methods were selected? To what extent was the therapist expected to act as an authoritative expert and to what extent as a friend? How *reactive* was the assumed role of the client?

2. A second question concerning mutual roles was: how *detached* was the therapeutic relationship? How much emotional involvement did both parties expect in it? To what extend was the therapist expected to respond to concrete needs of the client?

3. Concerning *assumed knowledge,* we were interested in the question of how much the therapist knew about the situation of the client (including the cultural background), and how important this knowledge was assumed to be. Conversely: how much did the client know about mental health care and what could be expected from this particular institution?

4. Concerning *motives,* we looked at the following questions: What was the client looking to get from the therapy? What did the therapist aim to provide? What were the motives of both of them for seeking or giving therapy?

1.2. Results

1.2.1. Views concerning cultural barriers to successful communication

Both therapists and clients tended towards the view that cultural differences existed, that they were important, but that they did not form a serious barrier in the interaction. This view was found in several different forms, but the general conclusion was clear. 'Culture' was a factor which operated *outside of* the therapeutic encounter: most respondents seemed to view it in terms of 'life-style', 'traditions' or 'conventions'. Differences in problem construction or 'explanatory models' were apparently not considered by most as a possible aspect of culture. As one therapist put it:

In therapy with refugees you have to deal with cultural differences, but these differences also play a role with other clients. Within the Dutch culture you'll find a lot of differences, for example on gender or, religion – it all makes a difference.

Most strikingly, the degree of satisfaction among both therapists and clients about the interaction was high – even, sometimes, when the client had been selected as an example of a 'difficult' or 'unsuccessful' interaction. Clients wanted above all to express *gratitude* and to praise the therapist for their insight and dedication. Without wishing to appear overly cynical, we should bear in mind here two things: firstly, that in any ongoing therapeutic relationship *transference* – often of the positive sort – plays a role; and secondly, that the clients were in a *dependent* relationship and unlikely to disclose their most critical thoughts, even in a supposedly confidential interview with a researcher. The positive views of the therapists may have to do with the fact that they have all gone out of their way to help refugees and have made something of a speciality of the work, including dealing with cultural differences. However, comparison of the interviews with therapists and clients revealed that the feeling of good communication was often no more than that: a feeling.

1.2.2. Views concerning the causes and nature of problems (explanatory models)

On this topic there were systematic divergences between therapists and clients. The refugees tended to relate their problems to external, concrete events, such as the political situation they had fled from, the experiences of violence and persecution they had been subjected to and their difficulties in gaining permission to stay in The Netherlands and in setting up a new life here. In contrast, therapists tended to define problems in terms of individual factors. They were aware of the 'objective' difficulties, but placed primary emphasis on the psychological reaction of the client to these difficulties. The concept of PTSD played a central role in their interpretations (though some therapists questioned whether the reactions to trauma should be regarded as 'pathological'). In some institutions, the use of such DSM categories is encouraged by the rule that clients cannot be treated unless they can be diagnosed with a recognized mental disorder. In this quotation, a refugee speaks about his therapist:

> *He helps me with my situation, I'm able to sleep better. I'm sick and he tells me about the process of having psychiatric complaints. I didn't have any rest and that's what I try to find here. And I also had political problems.*

When clients persisted in emphasizing the 'objective' problems and neglecting the 'subjective' ones, this tended to be interpreted by the therapist as a sign of resistance or psychic disturbance (for example 'paranoia' or 'over-dependency'). However, there were indications that in the course of therapy, many clients had shifted their views in the direction of those held by the therapists. In other words, they had adopted the therapist's explanatory model. Obviously, it is difficult for therapists to help clients to 'make sense' of their problems if both parties have fundamentally different notions about what 'making sense' involves. The problem is resolved, in these interactions, by the client adopting the notion of the therapist. As one of the participants in the workshop remarked, it would require a substantial change in the culture of mental health agencies to permit a shift in the opposite direction.

1.2.3. Views concerning the therapeutic interaction (the 'meta-contract')

As we saw in the previous section the meta-contract deals with *roles, knowledge* and *motives*. In relation to roles, we focused chiefly on *symmetry* and *detachment*.

(1) Most clients expected an asymmetrical relationship. The therapist is the one who knows what is wrong with them and their situation, not they themselves, and what should be done about it. The therapist should also sets the agenda for the interaction. As one refugee put it:

As a patient I can't tell which ideas I have about my problems. Only the doctor knows. Eventually I followed his advice and I must admit: it all helped. He (the therapist) was right in every sense.

Therapists, on the other hand, try in various ways to make the relationship more symmetrical, inviting the client to think together about the problems and their solution. When the client behaves passively ('reactively'), he or she runs the risk of being labeled over-dependent or immature. Even more serious labels are reserved for those who insist on the therapist helping more actively.

In our view, however, the differences which underlie this discrepancy are not so much a matter of individual personality as of cultural conventions. Many people from non-Western countries are simply not familiar with the 'rules of the game' which structure therapeutic interactions in the West. In De Swaan's terms (1982), they have not been sufficiently 'proto-professionalized'.

(2) With respect to *detachment* there were also divergent views. Clients often commented on the empathic, compassionate reactions of the therapist: these made them feel they were no longer completely on their own. After this woman's application for asylum was rejected, she said about the therapist:

She was almost as disappointed as I was. Not completely the same of course, but she was very compassionate.

However, many clients expected the therapist to be more involved: they found it difficult to accept that the therapist's dedication was only available at set times and by appointment. Such clients often perceived the behavior of the therapist as distant and controlled, lacking in spontaneity or emotional warmth. Others hoped that the therapist would offer advice, support and concrete help and were disappointed to be met with refusal. They wanted, sometimes explicitly, to be able to treat the therapist as a friend or a family member, who would help them with practical as well as emotional problems. In contrast, therapists expected refugees themselves to take responsibility for solving their own practical problems.

Here again, we see obvious differences in the 'meta-contract'. These differences sometimes led therapists – presumably unaware of their existence – to ascribe personality problems to the client. However, it was noteworthy that some therapists made an effort to adapt their approach to the expectations of the client. For example, some therapists mentioned that they accepted presents from refugees, though they would not do this with Dutch clients. Sometimes concrete help would also be given. The more committed therapists appeared to be wrestling with the problem of whether and how to bridge the gap between what clients expected and what they received.

(3) When we looked at *knowledge,* therapists appeared to have considerable knowledge about the situation of refugees in general, but sometimes this was accompanied by the attitude that it was not necessary to know the details of particular cases. Clients, on the other hand, were aware that they were in the dark about many aspects of mental health care and strongly criticized the adequacy of the information made available to them.

(4) The *motives* of many clients for starting or continuing the contact involved a need for human contact and understanding, which therapy to some extent met. Other clients appeared to be motivated to seek therapy not as an end in itself, but in the hope that through the therapist it would be possible to change their concrete situation (for example, to get better housing). The inability or unwillingness of the therapist to do this led to some resentment.

Concerning the therapists, those who had chosen to work with refugees were often concerned in other ways with human rights issues and/or politically active. In particular, they were very critical of the inhuman and stressful asylum procedures.

1.3. Discussion

When setting up this research, we had assumed that cultural differences would be likely to cause misunderstandings in the interactions between care-givers and refugees. This was in line with the thinking in that period, which we would now consider too 'culturalistic': it presumes that the differences between groups of users (e.g. refugees vs. native Dutch clients) are greater than the differences within each group. We also assumed the results would be to some extent generalizable – hopefully to other refugee and asylum seeker clients in therapy, perhaps even to those who never even come near mental health and social care services.

Our data are based on interviews concerning the interactions, rather than the interactions themselves. People can tell you what they do, but they may act quite differently in real life. That means that our conclusions could only be described in terms of views. Views concerning cultural barriers to successful communication, views concerning the causes and nature of problems and views concerning the therapeutic interaction.

The major shortcoming of this study, as it seems to us now, is the assumption that differences in 'culture' would be a major determinant of interactions between the caregivers and the clients in this study. Another weakness of the study is the focus on clients, to the exclusion of potential users who do not get therapy. As mentioned at the beginning of this chapter, the transference relationship between therapist and client may influence the remarks of both in unpredictable ways. In particular, the client may have feelings of loyalty to the therapist and for this reason be rather uncritical about the therapist's attitude and professional interventions.

Finally, what strikes us now, looking back at this study in the light of eight years of subsequent research with asylum seekers and refugees, is the large amount of theoretical baggage we brought to the study: our focus was mainly on testing the hypotheses we had in our heads, rather than learning to listen to the issues our respondents had in theirs.

1.4. Implications for service provision

The many discrepancies we found between the views of clients and therapists seem at odds with the optimistic statements both groups made about the ease with which cultural barriers could be overcome. Therapeutic interactions often seemed to be hampered by misunderstandings which could be traced to discrepancies between the culturally-determined expectations of the participants. 'Successful' interactions usually turned out to be those in which the client had adapted his or her expectations and problem definitions to those of the therapist. Therapists who wished to move in the reverse direction, for example by offering concrete help or emotional warmth, were afraid of coming in conflict with the culture of the institution within which they worked.

Clearly, it would not be possible to solve these problems simply by improving communication. A fundamental rethinking of the type of therapy appropriate to refugees is required, and it would appear that many therapists are aware of this. In particular, some refugee clients had difficulty with the 'meta-contract' underlying the therapeutic relationship, notably the expectation that the client is to a large extent responsible for finding the answers and that the relationship with the therapist ceases to exist, for practical purposes, at the end of the therapy session.

2. POLITICAL DIMENSIONS OF REFUGEES' PROBLEMS

2.1. Aim and method

This research (Kramer, 1999) focused on political aspects of refugees' problems and on the model used by therapists who, at present, seem to neglect or underestimate the importance of the political dimensions of the situation of asylum seekers and refugees. The reasons for this focus derive from the results of the research described above. Refugees mentioned political aspects of their problems, but they were not very explicit about them. Mental health services are aimed at individual and psychological dimensions of problems. The research set out to discover if and how social and political factors can be included in the explanatory models of service providers. To answer that question, I looked at examples from the women's movement and anti-psychiatry (Gijswijt-Hofstra & Porter, 1998).

The research was based on interviews with refugees, most of them non-users of services, and service providers, some of them refugees by origin. Specifically, the research group consisted of 37 persons, 22 of whom were refugees. About half of these had permission to stay in the Netherlands, the other half were still involved in the asylum procedure or had been turned down. Five refugees were working as therapists. Countries of origin were Iran, Iraq, former Yugoslavia, Chili and Eritrea. The research group was completed by 12 workers of the Refugee Council.

As a result of what we had learnt from the first study, we used a more dynamic model concerning differences in giving meaning to the situation. This was no longer based on cultural differences, but explored differences based upon a variety of subject positions and took changes over time into account.

2.2. Results

2.2.1. Opinions of refugees about the period before they flee to another country

Several respondents emphasized that refugees differ in a lot of ways. Countries of origin, varieties of political activity, being active or belonging to a group that is suppressed, the period of persecution and the personal characteristics of the refugee (including age, education and sex) can lead to big differences. That makes it difficult to talk about refugees as a group. As one Iranian refugee stated:

> *The political activities can be different. In the period of the cold war, refugees who were politically active fled to Europe. They belonged to the opposition. After the cold war, others fled. There was a high degree of control over daily life, due to Islamic*

laws. In both cases there are political reasons for fleeing the country but it's different.

Many respondents remembered the time in their own countries as a period of good health. Sometimes they felt bad about things that happened to them then, and these experiences sometimes came back after some time. The refugees who were not sure if they could stay in the Netherlands all stated that this uncertainty was a bigger problem than dealing with the memories or effects of the hardships they endured before or during their flight.

2.2.2 The period of the asylum procedure

There were many complaints about the juridical procedure and about the living conditions of the asylum seekers. The officials of the Immigration Board (IND), responsible for the juridical procedure, were sharply criticized. Respondents said they didn't have enough time, sometimes the translators are distrusted, refugees don't get the chance to tell their own story and some of them feel insulted. (Asylum procedures in the Netherlands were becoming become more restrictive during the period of the research.)

Complaints about the living conditions included lack of privacy, bad hygienic conditions, humiliations, being in a dependent position, too little responsibility, not enough access to medical help, problems in telecommunication and the spreading of family members over different asylum seekers' centers. There were many complaints about this period. One refugee said:

A lot of refugees come from dictatorships. They don't dare to speak up against the management of the asylum seeker's center. Sometimes they don't dare to speak about injustice in the care or support they get. They are afraid it will have a negative influence on their procedure. The complaints that get media attention are just a fraction of what is really going on.

2.2.3. The period after getting a status (residence permit)

To begin with, there is a great difference in the formal rights and responsibilities of refugees before and after they get a status. Before that moment, refugees are restricted in finding and accepting work, while educational possibilities are limited and sometimes not available. After getting a status, refugees are supposed to find a job and to speak Dutch, at least on an average level. A teacher of Dutch had this to say:

After they get a status, you notice how insecure people were. They are looking for new purposes in life, a new, safe haven. They still can't learn the language. They feel like stranded birds, still captives of their history.

There are a lot of problems in the period after getting a status. Some are seen as political problems, some as cultural conflicts. In the interviews the following problems were mentioned:

- Economic problems, the issues refugees share with other migrant groups: a higher level of unemployment, lower income levels and discrimination. Integration is often seen as a process in which refugees have to adapt Dutch norms and values. Refugees feel that they will always be seen as outsiders, even after naturalization and learning Dutch.

- Problems can arise with the education of children, due to cultural differences in the expectations parents have of the school system, the social roles they think are appropriate for the children and themselves, and the way the children are treated in schools and institutions. Sometimes these children are seen as disadvantaged, which leads to underestimating their potential.
- Often, there are concerns about family members who stayed behind, periods of mourning about the loss of the country of origin and living in exile, and problems as a reaction to incidents in the countries of origin (e.g. sickness or death of parents, political changes, etc.)
- Problems can also arise as a result of changes in gender roles and expectations, or as a result of the position of children and their ability to learn the language quicker than their parents.

2.2.4. The encounter with social workers and therapists

Several refugees said that they did not think that health care workers could understand what it means to live in a political system of repression or in conditions of war. They were reluctant to tell about these experiences. Refugees expected the health care workers to call attention to current social problems. One complained: "Social workers don't resist the policy, they accept the status quo and give us medicine."

Other problems concerned the accessibility of institutions for (mental) health and social care. The situation of refugees is sometimes quite dramatic when they come to services. A lot of refugees tell about periods of suicidal behavior as a reason for seeking help.

Problems were also mentioned with the treatment models, in particular the focus within therapy on the past and on 'working through' painful experiences. In communication with the caregivers, dealing with distance and affect was clearly an issue. Sometimes refugees expected therapists to take a familial role in being close to them (cf. the results of the first study).

The system of health care starts with an individual question for help. But problems of refugees are often very complex and have to do with all kind of circumstances. As a therapist said: "It is a great problem for refugees to divide their problems into all kind of sub-problems".

2.3. Discussion

This research focused on a particular issue in the situations and problem-constructions of refugees: the political aspects. To understand the political dimensions in the problems of refugees, I asked them to describe these in different periods in their lives. I also asked them about the confrontation with caregivers and the way political issues were handled by professional helpers.

The greatest weakness of this study is that what respondents say about the political aspects has nothing or little to do with how they approach caregivers, if they approach them at all. That makes this research the most theoretical of the four. It may be difficult to translate the results into therapeutic practice. Another pitfall is the small sample size and the individual differences in how problems are defined.

2.4. Implications for service provision

Refugees mention the political context of their problems and see this as a very important dimension of their difficulties in both the country of origin and the Netherlands. The political choices they made resulted in periods of violence and danger. Their political activities had an enormous impact on their lives and this is also true during the period of the asylum procedure. Refugees see this procedure as a political process and they feel they have little power to influence it. The procedures are unpredictable, hard to understand, take a lot of time and make refugees ill.

In the interaction between refugees and therapists, refugees expect that therapists should know about their background as political refugees. Therapists should be able to relate individual stories to structural factors such as politics, power, discrimination and integration. However, in the institutions for psycho-social help such as Community Mental Health Centers, this is a forgotten debate. The focus is on individual, psychological problems and individual processes of working through trauma-stories.

To help change the position of refugees in our society, therapists cannot maintain a neutral stance. They need become involved in 'group advocacy' and to seek cooperation with organizations for education, work and integration.

3. DIFFERENT MODELS FOR TREATING ASYLUM SEEKERS

3.1. Aim and method

After this more theoretical study, I felt the urge to go back to the notions we explored in the first project and to focus again on interactions between refugees or asylum seekers and their caregivers. Asylum seekers were a part of the research population in the first research, but this time I wanted to focus exclusively on this group. For them, social and political factors play an even more important role than for refugees. I also wanted to include the material of the interaction itself and that meant taping some sessions of caregivers with their asylum-seeker client. This research (Kramer, 2000) was done in three locations:

- a day care center for asylum seekers in Vught, The Netherlands;
- a treatment center for asylum seekers and refugees in Amsterdam (Pharos);
- the trauma center for victims of violence and torture in Cape Town, South Africa.

Only at one location (Amsterdam) was it possible to tape the direct interactions between asylum seekers and their caregivers. At the other locations the method of the first research was used, which meant holding interviews with therapists and clients. The sample consisted of twelve therapists and ten clients.

The data were collected on tape and transcribed fully, but we confine ourselves here to a summary of the main findings. A more detailed account of the interviews is given in the published versions of the research (Kramer, 2000a, 2000b)

3.2. Results

- The explanatory model of the day care center can be described as a trauma model. Asylum seekers' complaints are interpreted as reactions to traumatic events, which have led to weakening of the core beliefs of trust and security. The main aim of the treatment is to restore these core beliefs. The trauma model contains all the elements of a medical model. The assessment of problems is on an individual level, using psychiatric classification and diagnostic tools; complaints are identified and treatment is focused on their reduction.
- The therapists of the Pharos Foundation in Amsterdam adopt a position between two extremes. They try to focus on the combination of trauma, displacement, and insecurity in daily life and loss as an explanatory model for their clients' problems. The therapists try to understand the clients' experiences in their social context, while considering the possibilities of altering the current situation as well as helping the clients find their own coping strategies.
- The mental health care in the trauma center for victims of violence and torture in Cape Town is highly politicized. Collective and political dimensions are clearly represented in the explanatory models of the therapists. Therapists identified their clients as survivors of human rights violations. They use advocacy and empowerment as concepts.

3.3. Discussion

The interactions between mental health care workers and clients showed that on a local level one can see the effect of different treatment models, including the explanation adopted for the problems and the view of how these problems could be solved. Mental health care professionals always have to deal with the dynamic between the individual and the social context. The choice of model can significantly affect client-professional interactions. In a model, the focus can be on individual aspects – the medical or psychological consequences of traumatic experiences – or on the collective and political aspects of a client's sense of isolation or deprivation.

The main drawback of this project was that the method used was very time-consuming. The results are based on a small sample but show similar patterns as in the first study. It would have been preferable to do the observations in the first phase, but organizations did not give permission to tape these interviews. A great deal of time is required to become familiar with the organizations and professionals under study.

3.4. Implications for service provision

The fact that a part of the data is based on the real interactions between therapists and clients, not just on their opinions about the interactions, enhances the value of the results of this study. This comparison across three locations, one outside Europe, shows that one can map explanatory models by interviewing and/or observing clients and therapists. Therapists differ in the degree to which they take contextual and political aspects of the situation of their clients into account.

4. MAKING SENSE OF EXPERIENCE

4.1. Aim and method

Learning from the shortcomings of the previous studies, *Making sense of experience: research on patterns in giving meaning to the situation and coping of asylum seekers* (Kramer et al., 2003; see also Van Dijk et al., 2002; Bala & Kramer, 2004) also attempted to get closer to the perspective of asylum seekers. The background to the project was formed by a change in Dutch health care policy regarding asylum seekers. With effect from January 2000, mental health care for asylum seekers became the responsibility of regular service providers and costs were covered by a special form of health insurance. The company providing this insurance set aside part of funds it received from the Dutch Government for innovative projects and the development of expertise in this area. The present study was financed from this source in order to gain insight into the way asylum seekers experience their situation and the patterns of coping they adopted. Four researchers (a cross-cultural psychologist, a psychologist/ psychotherapist, a medical anthropologist and a medical doctor) developed a qualitative, exploratory research design and gathered relevant data . The research took place between February 2001 and July 2002 in one of the 150 centers for asylum seekers in the Netherlands.

The researchers decided not to use standardized instruments and questionnaires in order to focus on the unique experiences of the refugees living in centers for asylum seekers. Without intruding on the refugees' stories, the researchers relied on theoretical concepts concerning the construction of meaning (Bruner, 1990; De Ruijter, 1996), coping (Lazarus & Folkman, 1984), and the search for significance in times of stress (Pargament, 1997) as a general frame for the research. The researchers wanted to develop a model based on the observations and definitions that the refugees introduced themselves, within their own frame of reference.

During the period of observations and interviews, the researchers used a small room, a former shed intended to accommodate one person, in an asylum seekers center. They thus obtained first-hand experience of what it was like to live in such centers. Observations, open and semi-structured interviews, in individual or group settings were used to collect information. Most of the contacts continued after the first encounter and the researchers could discuss intensively the topics which concerned the inmates of the asylum center. The research focused on the issues which the asylum seekers themselves found important.

Out of 285 persons living in this asylum center, the researchers spoke with 36 men and 14 women between 12 and 54 years of age. These respondents illustrated the diversity of the refugee population living in the center for asylum seekers.

4.2. Results

The interviews with the asylum seekers revealed five relevant domains of their lives: *social contacts, activities, perspective, self-image* and *balance*. These were the main themes we found in the way refugees define themselves and look for meaning in everyday life. We assume that the same domains will also be found in other groups, but for people living in the asylum center three of the five domains were significantly restricted.

(1) Many refugees reported that they felt lonely. Their *social contacts* were limited, they missed member(s) of their family, most of them have had minimal contact with other residents and they rarely had any contact with Dutch people outside the center for asylum seekers. Refugees who managed to build significant relationships in these difficult conditions were in the minority.

(2) Refugees have limited opportunities to engage in meaningful *activities* because asylum seekers in the Netherlands are prohibited from having a regular job. They are allowed by law to work only twelve weeks a year, in a limited range of jobs (mainly seasonal labor). Language is another obstacle to social activities, presenting a psychological barrier to getting in contact with Dutch citizens. Despite these restrictions, some of the refugees are creative in finding meaningful activities, opening a bar in the recreation room, organizing creative activities for the children or delivering newspapers during a few hours a day.

(3) *Perspective* refers to the refugees' attitude toward the asylum procedure, often experienced as blocked because of the procedure's long-lasting uncertainly and unpredictable outcome. But perspective also refers to the goals and objectives people have for the rest of their lives. The researchers found that many of the residents had lost faith in the future or could only think about the present and perhaps a day beyond. Few of them managed to think about the future within a broader perspective.

(4) The restrictions on these three domains can have an effect on the refugees' *self image*, the way refugees experience and define themselves and how they are perceived by others. Many of the residents consider themselves to be second-rate citizens, worthless individuals, reduced to seeking asylum in a foreign land. They start to feel ill or depressed. Few of them manage to find inspiration in new contacts or experiences; others seem to wait, holding on to their former experiences and self-image.

(5) *Balance*, the last domain, includes a general evaluation that a person makes about him- or herself in the present situation. It is an all-encompassing attitude that includes the other domains. Balance is a dynamic process that changes continuously over time according to the experiences that influence the way people think and feel. For most residents, life in a center for asylum seekers has become senseless. They resist and dislike the situation they find themselves in; some residents are more profoundly affected and begin doubting the meaningfulness of life. Only a minority of the asylum seekers defined their new experiences as positive challenges.

These five domains are sufficiently distinctive to cover and describe different parts of the experiences of refugees in centers for asylum seekers. The researchers then examined differences within each of the five domains, to identify patterns of coping with life in a center for asylum seekers. We found four different styles or patterns of coping: *the drifter, the hibernator, the fighter and the explorer*. People usually cannot be reduced to one single pattern, rather they use various coping styles in combination and context bound.

(1) The pattern of the *drifter* is recognized in refugees who believe that they have no way to influence the outcome of events. They drift in directions controlled by forces beyond their control. This position is illustrated by the following remarks by a woman refugee:

I'm tired, so tired. One day I'll kill myself. I don't want anything anymore, no status, nothing. The first months I only slept. I asked myself: what am I doing here? I have headaches, my stomach aches and I have problems with my head. Why do I have to wait so long? It drives me mad. Why do the Netherlands need so many mad people?

(2) For those whose behavior resembles the pattern of *hibernator*, time seems to be frozen. They wait for the future to arrive, in order to go on with their lives. Refugees using this pattern live in the present but cling to what they had and who they were in the past.

I ignore many things. So many fights about small things (with fellow residents). I ignore them. I believe in God and he supports me.

(3) *Fighters* are active, on the lookout for ways and means to change their situation. They focus more on the external world and may be involved in all kinds of contacts and activities, some with only an instrumental purpose, and others with a larger scope involving the struggle for rights and justice. As one woman said:

Don't wait for others to do something for you before you do it yourself. So many people here know nothing about the procedures For example, how to get a house when you get a status. You should ask for information and act upon it.

(4) The pattern of the *explorer* is recognized in few refugees who are open to new options and opportunities. They manage to preserve their positive self-image at least temporarily and/or in some areas of functioning. They are active and flexible, changing their strategies to achieve certain goals or even changing the goals themselves. A male refugee:

I know a lot of people outside the center. One of them offered me a job, at his farm and although I'm not used to physical labor, I took it. The week after his neighbor asked me to help him too but now I knew what I could ask and he didn't accept my offer. But I'm sure I'll find other ways of earning some money."

4.3. Discussion

Three dichotomies were found to explain the refugees' different styles of coping: chaos versus coherence, internal versus external locus of control and low versus high degree of flexibility. These concepts discriminated the patterns of coping amongst asylum seekers.

Those who felt the highest level of chaos could be described as *drifters*. When people experience an external locus of control, they are seen as *hibernators*. (We are talking here about perceived control; in reality, of course, asylum seekers in fact have very little control over their situation.) The third concept, flexibility, distinguishes *fighters* from *explorers*. Explorers are more keen to change their strategies to obtain certain goals or to change the goals themselves.

Using these three concepts helped explain the different styles of coping, but it raised a whole series of new questions. One is the question of continuity. Were the coping strategies found among the asylum seekers in the Netherlands the same as they had used in the country of origin? Another question is: how and under which conditions do patterns of coping change?

This kind of research is, again, very time-consuming and not easy to fund. Another pitfall in using this approach, which avoids using pre-selected categories, is that it tends to become an analysis of how people in general give meaning to life.

4.4. Implications for service provision

The implications of these findings were worked out in a subsequent implementation project, financed by the same health insurance company and carried out within a mental health care service provider. In this project, the results of the research were presented to a specialized team of mental health care workers who had been dealing with this target group since 1995. This team consisted of two doctors, a psychiatrist and two psychiatric nurses.

In the first part of the project, members of the team were interviewed separately about the special features of working with asylum seekers. They mentioned the intense stresses originating before or during the flight, as well as the difficult living conditions in the centers and the stress caused by asylum policies and procedures. Working with this group requires more time for establishing good communication and building up trust. Against the background of enormous and sometimes insoluble real-life problems, mental health workers concentrate on the small steps which can be taken to make life more livable. Interviews with nine clients were undertaken to obtain the users' side of the picture.

In the next stage of the project, the mental health workers were familiarized with the results of the research project *Making sense of experience* and asked to relate the categories emerging from this study to their own clients. They found this exercise useful. Subsequently, a team of preventive health workers joined the project and was also introduced to the results of the study.

The preliminary results of this project suggest that mental health workers, even those working in the area of prevention, remain largely oriented towards a goal of symptom reduction rather than changing the ways in which clients attempt to cope with their situation. The research project showed much variation in the coping styles adopted by asylum seekers, but there do not seem to be at present many interventions which address this question.

5. CONCLUSION: HOW CLOSE CAN ONE GET?

The four phases in the research on asylum seekers and refugees can be seen as a progression towards getting as close as possible to the perspective of the users of mental health services. This involved also analyzing the perspectives of non-clients. When we review the pitfalls and conclusions of the different researches, some general lessons for mental health care for asylum seekers and refugees can be drawn.

5.1. Power and a dominant discourse

Looking back at the first phase of the research, we were quite aware of the power imbalance between refugees and their therapists. As in probably all enduring contacts between clients and therapists, the one who is more independent than the other can define the 'rules of the game'. For a researcher it is important not to stop asking questions when one finds clients who are satisfied. One should be aware of the side-effects, of the underlying expectations and the desperate situation clients can be in. When badly in need of contact, people sometimes accept almost any source of advice.

The experience therapists have with their clients has only a small effect on the discourse on refugees in Western society, which is formed by media, political debates, sociological shifts and medical belief systems. All these factors play a role in determining how the problems of refugees and asylum seekers are constructed. It is worth taking this wider discourse into account when one is trying to make sense of the experience of the asylum seekers themselves.

5.2. The world outside the consulting room

From the second study onwards, respondents were no longer selected on the basis of being the client of a mental health care worker. This probably gives us better access to the meanings which asylum seekers and refugees ascribe to the situation they are living in, the difficulties they face and the kinds of problems which may lead them to seek (or be recommended) professional help. Research carried out using 'clinical' samples should always be replicated with the general population, because unsuspected differences may exist between service users and non-users.

5.3. Life is multi-faceted

As was shown in all the studies discussed above, but perhaps most clearly in the last one, to really take into account the perspective of refugees or asylum seekers one has to be open to very different ways of conceptualizing situations. It is important not to reduce the problems of asylum seekers or refugees to medical or psychological dimensions. We started these researches with a lot of theoretical assumptions about cultural differences. Such theoretical preoccupations can get in the way of having a truly open mind towards the reality. To get closer to the situation of asylum seekers and refugees and they way they experience it, researchers need to take time and devote a lot of energy to building up trust. This trust also needs to be built up between the researcher and the institutions involved: this is illustrated by the reluctance of organizations to permit tape recordings of therapeutic interactions. Asylum seekers and refugees illustrate that giving meaning to life is a multi-faceted and a multi-phased process.

REFERENCES

Bala, J. & Kramer, S.A. (2004) Managing uncertainty: coping styles of refugees in a Western country. *Intervention 2*, 33-42.

Boomstra, R. & Kramer, S.A. (1997) *Cultuurverschillen in interacties tussen hulpverleners en vluchtelingen.* Utrecht: ISOR.

Broekx, G., Knoppers, M & van Tienhoven, H. (1980) *De buitenlandse patiënt.* Bunnik: Buro Voorlichting Gezondheidszorg Buitenlanders.

Bruner, J. (1990) *Acts of meaning.* Cambridge: Harvard University Press.

De Ruijter, A. (1996) Betekenisconstructie en sturing in een complexe wereld. In Gastelaars, M. & Hagelsteijn, G. (eds.), *Management of meaning.* Utrecht: ISOR.

De Swaan, A. (1982) *De mens is de mens een zorg.* Amsterdam: Meulenhoff.

Gijswijt-Hofstra, M. and Porter, R. (eds.) (1996). *Cultures of psychiatry and mental health care in postwar Britain and the Netherlands.* Amsterdam: Rodopi.

Kleinman, A. (1981) *Patients and healers in the context of culture: an exploration of the borderland between anthropology, medicine and psychiatry.* Berkeley, CA: University of California Press.

Kramer, S.A. (1999) *Het psychologiseren van politieke ervaringen.* Utrecht: ISOR

Kramer, S.A. (2000a) *Gezocht: asiel en hulp.* Utrecht: ISOR.

Kramer, S.A. (2000b) Doctors or political activists? Mental health care workers in interaction with asylum seekers. In: M. Gastelaars (ed.), *On Location: The relevance of the 'here' and 'now' in organizations.* Maastricht: Shaker Publishing.

Kramer, S.A., Bala, J., Van Dijk, R. & F. Öry (2003) *Making sense of experience.* Utrecht: USBO.

Kramer, S.A. (2004) Hoe geven asielzoekers betekenis aan hun ervaringen? *Cultuur Migratie Gezondheid 1*, 34-48.

Lazarus, R.S. & Folkman, S. (1984) Coping and adaptation. In Gentry, W.D. (ed.), *Handbook of Behavioral Medicine.* New York: Guilford Press

Pargament, K. (1997) *The psychology of religion and coping, theory, research, practice.* New York: Guilford Press.

Richters, A. (1996) *Medische en psychiatrische antropologie: een terreinverkenning.* In De Jong, J. & Van den Berg, M. (eds.), *Transculturele psychiatrie en psychotherapie. Handboek voor hulpverlening en beleid.* Amsterdam/Lisse: Swets & Zeitlinger.

Rommetveit, R. (1974) *On message structure: a framework for the study of language and communication.* New York: Academic Press.

Young, A. (1979) Internalizing and externalizing medical belief systems: An Ethiopian example. *Social Science and Medicine 10*, 147-156

Van der Veer, G. (1992/1998) *Counselling and therapy with refugees.* New York: Wiley.

Van Dijk, R., Bala, J., Kramer, S. and Öry, F. (2002) "Now we have lost everything". Asylum seekers and their experiences with health care. *Medische Antropologie 13*, 284-301.

9. KURDISH WOMEN REFUGEES
Obstacles and opportunities

Choman Hardi[1]

This paper is mainly based on my research findings with Kurdish women refugees and my work facilitating creative writing workshops with refugee women in Britain. I have also drawn on my own experiences as a refugee woman in the UK and my knowledge of the Kurdish community. It is divided into three parts. I will first talk about the immediate problems that refugee women face as a result of seeking asylum and then go on to talk about what I call further problems for refugee women. In the third part I will talk about ways of empowerment for refugee women.

From my own experience of exile and the Kurdish community in Britain I have found that the problems that result from migration do not end. They merely change shape and scope. As time goes on things do indeed become easier, and some of the women I have interviewed are great examples of resilience and success. Still, as women who have come from one community to live in another, we have to keep negotiating our two worlds if we are to fit the different roles we find ourselves occupying. Those who fail to handle this delicate position may put their own lives in danger. On the evening of October 12th 2002 the seventeen-year-old Kurdish girl, Heshu Yunis, was killed by her father in London in an act of honor killing. Heshu was probably too young to realize the dangers she was putting herself into. She probably did not have anyone who could advise and protect her. I thus dedicate this paper to her, and to women like her who carry the burden of living between two cultures.

1. IMMEDIATE PROBLEMS FOR REFUGEE WOMEN

When arriving in exile and seeking asylum, a person's world is turned upside down. She is suddenly in a situation where she has no control over her environment. She is without her friends and family and finds herself in a new setting where she does not speak the language and is not familiar with the system and the culture. On arrival she may find that her past education and experience are redundant in the new country and she has to start everything from scratch. In this sense, the immediate feeling a person experiences is being overwhelmed. The factors that contribute to this feeling are

---

[1] Choman Hardi, European Centre for Migration and Social Care Studies, University of Kent, Canterbury, UK.

uncertainty about her fate in the new country (the asylum application), having to cope with loss and the need to adapt to a great number of changes. I shall talk about each of these in turn and provide examples from my research.

1.1. Uncertainty about the future

Once a person seeks asylum, she will have no control over the events following this moment. Until the asylum application is processed and the person's legal status is determined she feels uncertain about the future. She may be in suspense for years, her asylum application may be refused and she may even be deported. Living with these thoughts contributes to a general feeling of malaise and gloom. This uncertainty concerns not just her legal status, but also her entitlement to benefits and accommodation - and her life in general.

While the asylum application is being processed, the person is supported by NASS (National Asylum Support Service) and when a decision is reached NASS support and accommodation will stop. She will then have to apply for housing and support from the local council. This state of suspense influences people's plans for the future; some feel they cannot settle down in their current accommodation because they might be moved again.

Halima[2], who is in her early sixties, has been living in Hull for three and a half years and only recently she was granted Exceptional Leave to Remain. She has had a stroke in Turkey, while she was on her way to the UK, and is still affected by it. Halima has been living with her ten-year-old daughter in a flat provided by NASS. There was no telephone in her flat and three years down the line she still does not have one. When I asked her why, she told me it was because she didn't know what will happen to her and her daughter. She didn't feel settled enough to get a phone line although this has implied more isolation for her.

While waiting for the asylum application to be processed, a person is not allowed to work. This also influences people's lives: they end up waiting at home, not having anything else to do but to think about their situation.

Shireen, a young woman in her mid-twenties who has been waiting two years to hear about her asylum application, told me that being refused is better than not knowing what is going on. When you are refused, she said, "at least you know where you stand". Back home, Shireen used to be a very active young woman, acting and directing plays as well as being a presenter on one of the Kurdish satellite channels. Now, because her legal status is not determined, she cannot work. She is entitled to two half days of learning English and this has left her with plenty of time to reflect on her past life and feel sorry for herself. She keeps thinking that she should have stayed back home no matter what.

---

[2] First names used to refer to respondents are fictitious. Names are printed bold the first time they occur.

1.2. Loss

The losses a person experiences when leaving her home behind are many. They range from losing meaningful relationships to loss of social and material status, employment and relevant qualifications, and in general loss of what Hartman named the "average expectable environment" (Hartman, 1964, cited in Espin, 1992), in which the person knows her environment, is familiar and confident about where she is, is surrounded by the familiar smells, sounds, and tastes, and practices her daily routines. The losses are highly disorientating for the individual, leaving her confused and in a state of grief. I shall give a few examples from my research.

Salma is a woman in her mid-thirties who arrived in London in 1998. She suffered from depression on and off for the first three years until her husband was able to join her in London. She spoke about her loss of a support network and how it has affected her. She was a housewife back home, living close to her family, and was very well supported by her sister, mother and husband. Her husband did the shopping for her and her sister and mother helped her raising her sons, so that she "never felt she had two young kids". Suddenly on her own, without knowing anyone or speaking the language, she was crying a lot and feeling depressed. She developed many health problems which she believes were caused by her general unhappiness and loneliness.

Rezan spoke about the loss of material status which influences her social life and happiness. She was a lawyer back home, married to a businessman. When talking about where she lives in Hull, she mentioned how at home her kitchen alone "was the size of this house". She talked about "the shrinking of surfaces" in the UK which she believed influenced her life, in particular her social life. Rezan recalled the large social gatherings back home and how in her new accommodation she cannot invite "a couple of families around at the same time"; she felt very much restricted by her new setting.

Shireen used to be a famous and well respected actress and TV presenter: she spoke about loss of social status. After recalling how she was always recognized wherever she went back home and how everyone admired and respected her, she felt that she has become 'a nobody' in London. She said that it is only because her family are supporting her and understand what she is going through that she is surviving.

1.3. Adaptational tasks

The adaptational tasks include becoming familiar with a new physical environment which may be much larger than the one a person is used to, learning a new language, understanding and accepting the new culture in order to adjust her behavior accordingly, coping with culture shock, rebuilding a support network, needing to re-quality in some cases, and possibly coping with discrimination and racism.

Mani spoke about the difficulties of getting used to London. She was a well established lawyer back home and arrived in the UK in her late twenties having recently got divorced. She arrived with her younger sister and sought advice from someone she knew. Mani found the changes so overwhelming that she put all her trust in this person and ended up taking the wrong choices. One of the things that made her feel overwhelmed was the vastness of London. She found tubes and trains too complicated and for four months she "did not know how to use the tube or trains", she felt "blind and hopeless". This in turn made her feel very much dependant on her friend who used her and misguided her. She keeps wishing she was a bit more brave and had more faith in herself when she arrived.

Tanya *came with her husband and two children not speaking any English. This meant that she was afraid to go out alone and wouldn't 'answer the door or go out' on her own. She started college in the first month to learn English, but she 'kept hoping that no one will ask' her 'any questions or try to talk to' her. Not speaking the language made her lose faith in herself and it took her six months to be able to go out on her own and have faith in herself again. Only then was she able to do the shopping and go to the doctor alone and later she was able to answer the phone.*

Some women talked about the difficulties they encountered while trying to find a job in the UK.:

For **Dila***, who came in her late forties in 1997 having worked in her home country as a teacher and for Save the Children, finding work has proved extremely difficult. She has become clinically depressed a number of times and believes that '70%' of her depression is due to not having work. She used to be 'very capable and brave' but her depression has made her 'hopeless'. Dila believes not being able to get a job is partly due to her age and also due to her not speaking fluent English. When she arrived, Dila was 'depressed' about the cultural differences she found. These differences made her reflect on her home culture and compare and choose values from each. Recently she has started learning English again and has been feeling more hopeful. She aims to speak fluent English and get a degree and eventually find a job.*

But these are only some of the immediate problems that refugee women face. Later, even when some initial problems have been resolved, they may face different kinds of problems. That is, even when they are granted asylum, learn the language, become familiar with their environment and the culture, find jobs and recreate a support network, they may face other difficulties. The latter may include: maintaining family coherence in the face of possible role reversals and intergenerational conflict, mothers struggling to pass on their religion and culture to their children, younger women being in conflict with their families because of adopting new identities, living with discrimination and racism in their environment, and the psychological impact of becoming members of an ethnic minority group when they were members of the majority in their homeland. All these factors also contribute to low self-esteem and impose restrictions on the realization of their goals, their happiness, and satisfaction with their lives. I will now go on to talk about some of these problems.

2. FURTHER PROBLEMS FOR REFUGEE WOMEN

The problems associated with migration have no clearly defined end-point. So far I have spoken only of the first phase of these problems, but even when a person's legal status is determined and she settles down in the host country, there are problems of a different kind. Migration can lead to major changes in women's lives and this leads to other complications. Some of the changes may be negative like grieving for the lost life, friends and position, but some are positive such as having more opportunities, studying and working. Below I will talk about some of the ways that these changes can influence, change and sometimes reverse the power relationships a woman has with her immediate surroundings. A woman's role in her family may change, and the balance of power in the family may change. I will talk about these changes for three groups of women.

2.1. Married women

Migration can influence the status of men and women in different ways. A man may lose his job and therefore his role as the breadwinner, while a woman, who may have been a housewife, may find work and become more active outside the realm of her household. This is particularly true in the case of women who have arrived in exile before their husbands. They have had an opportunity to learn the language, settle down and sometimes find work before their husbands arrive. This can lead to 'role reversal', where the woman becomes a breadwinner and the man a house-husband. Some men find this more difficult to cope with than others. Some can take pride in their wife's success, yet still feel sorry for themselves, and this influences their relationship. Others feel extremely jealous and want to restrict their wives and prevent them from progressing.

In his home country Tanya's husband was a well-established doctor. Now, however, he does not work and spends most of his time at home. Tanya, on the other hand, went through a stage of being scared to go out on her own and losing confidence in herself when she first arrived in the UK. Six years on, she has raised four children (two of them step-children) and her English has improved a great deal. She has been taking many courses and wants to work. Tanya's ambitions have made her husband insecure and she believes he uses the children to 'tie her hand's. His way of defending himself is by not helping her around the house. When I first met them, he had picked up his young son from school and said that the teacher nearly didn't allow him to take the child because she had never seen him before. Tanya thus has to cope with looking after the house and her four children as well as doing her courses and training, without any help from her husband.

Salma used to be a housewife back home and arrived at the UK with her two sons three years before her husband. Salma found life extremely difficult in London, she had never even done shopping back home, her husband used to do the outside work for her. She was depressed for a long time and kept thinking if only her husband was around, she could rely on him a little and rest. She found looking after her two sons alone, when she didn't speak the language and was not familiar with the system, exhausting. Eventually her husband arrived but by this time because she spoke some English and he didn't, he became another burden for her.

When I met her she showed me all the forms and documents she had to complete on his behalf. This has been very difficult for both of them, for Salma, her husband is not the man she could rely on and for her husband because he feels useless and dependant on his wife.

2.2. Mothers

Migration can change the role of women as mothers. If previously mothers were the main caregiver for their children within a circle of others, in exile they become the sole caregiver. This includes the practical aspects of child caring as well as the tasks of socialization and transforming culturally important codes to their children. This shift from being an important figure in a network of caregivers for children to being the only responsible figure creates great pressure for these women.

Mothers worry about transforming cultural important values to their children. Dasgupta (1998) in her study with Asian Indians pointed out that the task of maintaining traditions and identity has historically been placed on women's shoulders. As guardians of traditions, women struggle to translate culturally important values to their children. Soon after their children start school, the women realize that their children are becoming anglicized very quickly: as their English improves, their Kurdish deteriorates. As they settle down in school and get familiar with the new codes of conduct, their cultural values start shifting towards western ones. The mother tongue can be a problem for some Kurdish children who live in the West. Many families take their children to weekend schools in order to learn how to read and write in Kurdish. Four of the seven women whose children are of schooling age take their children to weekend Kurdish schools.

Layla's sons are now both in their early twenties, they speak fluent Kurdish and know how to read and write in that language. During one of our conversations she told me how difficult it has been to try to convey some values of the Kurdish culture to her children. She took her children to the Kurdish school every Saturday for a few years. This meant that she had to give up her days off, days when she could have socialized, in order to make sure her children spoke proper Kurdish and were able to read and write. The school was also good because they had a music teacher who taught them Kurdish hymns and they were able to mingle with other Kurdish children and meet other adults.

*Salma and **Zara** are doing the same thing now. I met both of them in the Kurdish school that is managed by one of the Kurdish community centers. The women come to the location, many of them stay around all day, talking to each other, helping each other do their homework and generally chatting and having a laugh while their children learn Kurdish. Some families come and drop their children in the morning and pick them up in the afternoon.*

When I first met Salma and Zara I asked them why they thought it necessary to bring their children to the school. They both agreed that if they didn't, their children would end up talking solely in English. Tanya's children also went to a Kurdish school. In order to make sure the children learnt Kurdish, their father (who is a doctor by profession) started teaching in the Saturday school. The older two are both capable of writing letters in Kurdish to their uncles and aunts.

Zara discovered that there are many children's books in English, so she contacted her family and they sent her a few Kurdish story books. All four families also have satellite TV and have access to Kurdish channels. Although this is partly so that they can be aware of what is going on back home, is also intended to help their children keep in touch with their home culture. The satellite channels target Kurdish children in Europe and have lengthy children's programs starting around five in the afternoon. The programs include Kurdish cartoons, songs for children, stories, and a daily lesson on the alphabet. Both Zara and Salma believed the satellite channels have been great help in keeping their children interested in Kurdish as a language and a culture.

Another area for potential problems is religion. Families that want to bring up their children as Muslims may have a lot of difficulty in a non-Islamic culture. For example, most children very much enjoy Christmas because it is celebrated on a large scale around them and there is a lot of hype around celebrating it. However, they do not think much of Eid or any of the Islamic celebrations, because in school and their environment no one else may be celebrating it. Many of the women who took part in this research celebrate Christmas because they don't want their children to be deprived of it. Tanya's children have also taken part in the plays that are set up around Christmas about Jesus and Mary. The parents go to see their children and encourage them because they don't want them to feel left out. At the same time, celebrating Eid has become more difficult. Traditionally on Eid all the family gets together, wearing their new clothes, cooking for breakfast, kissing each other and the children receiving *jejnana* (money to buy whatever they like). On these days there are also fun-fairs in every neighborhood, and neighbors and relatives visit each other. It is hard to keep the traditions going when the large family is not there anymore and the fun-fairs and neighborhoods are not the same.

Nevertheless, many of the Kurdish families keep up the routine of celebrating Eid, cooking a feast for breakfast and instead of visiting each other, sending their Eid greetings by telephone. The satellite channels are a great help again because special programs are put on at this time and the images of people celebrating Eid back home are brought to everyone's homes. Some families insist that their children learn to pray and read the Qura'n. In such cases the parents find an Imam who may be able to educate their children. None of the women I have interviewed have gone to these lengths. They do, however, want their children to think of themselves as Muslim, know about the general rules, not eat pork and celebrate the Islamic occasions. Tanya pointed this out when she said:

> They know we are Muslim, they know about the Islamic fiestas. They know some of the short verses of Qura'n. At the Kurdish school they were even taught how to do ablution before prayer. They also know that Muslims shouldn't drink alcohol. In the last few years more members of the family have come over so we get together, the children speak in Kurdish, say *Eid mubarak.*

Some mothers are also greatly concerned about their children's sexuality. This is particularly true if a family have daughters. Within the Kurdish community there is no shame if a male child has a girl-friend, but an important taboo is broken if a female child is perceived to have a relationship or be sexually active. I shall come back to this point in the next section.

The issue of language and Kurdish identity becomes even more acute for people who intermarry.

Lana, who doesn't have any children yet and is married to an Englishman, talked about wanting her child to be Kurdish and how difficult that may be. She pointed out that she would rather have her children looked after by a Kurdish woman, preferably her own mother, than send them to a nursery in the UK. This is particularly because, in her own words, "my language is very important to me; I want my child to speak my language". She also wants her children to have a similar upbringing to herself, inheriting the same values.
Lana then talked about the difficulties of raising a child the Kurdish way. "This is a difficult society to bring up children in", she said. This is particularly because the children "will be leaning towards Western culture" rather than Kurdish. Lana does not want her children to take on some of the codes of this society. She does not, for example, want them to have boy-friends when they are too young, to smoke or take drugs. Lana also is very close to her family and likes her children to value family and respect the elderly, which seem to be missing in the British culture. Although Lana has married an Englishman, she said that she wanted her children to be "Kurdish first and then English", with a Kurdish name. The main reason for this, according to Lana, is the fact that she does not have her own nation state and in this sense she needs a stronger identity than her husband. This seemed to me to be making a very important point: the weaker identity has a stronger will to survive. To her, Kurdish identity is endangered but English identity is not:

> He doesn't need an identity, he has his powerful country, I don't, I don't have an identity as such so I need to have children and raise them Kurdish. I feel strongly about these issues, he doesn't that much.

Lana is particularly happy that her husband understands what she wants and accepts it. The issue of maintaining a strong identity is more important in her community, because their identity has constantly being threatened throughout history. This may be another reason why mixed marriages are frowned on. When I myself got married to an English man there was a lot of disapproval from the community. Some people had said what a shame, from such a patriotic father comes a daughter that abandons her Kurdish identity. This is almost more important than religious differences for many individuals within the community. The pressure is also more on young women because they are expected to continue and transfer identity and cultural values.

2.3. Younger women

Younger women may be pressurized from their ethnic community to maintain traditional values and culture. In this sense, women are seen as keepers of tradition. Nazli Kibria in a study with Vietnamese women says: "women experience singular conflicts that generate from contradiction between patriarchal family ideologies and personal bids for autonomy" (Kibria, 1987, 1993, cited in Dasgupta, 1998). In this sense women who may be critical of some aspects of their birth-culture and want to adopt some western values, will be opposed by their own families as well as other members of the ethnic community, leading to stress and division of loyalty. Wanting to adopt more egalitarian gender roles, for example, thus leads to other complications. This becomes more important in the light of the fact that there may be opportunities that refugee women might want to make use of, for example in the areas of employment and education.

From my own experience within the Kurdish community I know that problems arise when younger women want to go to a university in a different city from where their parents live. Letting their daughter go to live in residential halls where girls and boys live together terrifies some families. They worry that their daughter might become sexually active, or might end up marrying someone from a different religion and culture. Families and communities work harder at disciplining their daughters and controlling them. In a study carried out with South Asian communities Mani (1992, p. 13, cited in Dasgupta, 1998) suggests:

> .... the fear of dating that consumes many.. families is primarily a fear of women dating. Although many parents worry about interracial marriage for what it might imply for them in old age, there is little attempt to control men's sexuality. Women, meanwhile, are quite frequently policed with the stick of tradition: it is women who are called on to preserve the ways of the old country

Although Mani's study is concerned with South Asian immigrant families it is also relevant to refugee communities, for both communities have the same concerns about women and traditions. The taboos surrounding these issues and the division that these women experience leads to higher levels of anxiety compared to men (Dasgupta, 1998).

In the Kurdish community it is generally acceptable for a young man to have a girl-friend, drink alcohol, go to clubs and live alone before he gets married. However, Kurdish girls are not allowed a fraction of these rights. For my research I tried to interview some girls aged between 16 and 20 to find out about their problems and concerns, but I was not able to. The families of the girls did not agree for them to take part. One woman very openly told me that her daughter was young, she might have made some mistakes and they don't want anyone to know about them. This is also a form of control imposed by the families to stop the girls expressing themselves because the community is constantly worried about gossip.

Henar, who is the youngest participant to my research, is in her early twenties. She believes that gossip is much worse in the Kurdish community in Britain. This is particularly because "back home there were groups of families who knew each other and only mingled with each other": this meant that the families socialized with other families who had similar values. But 'in exile people don't have that choice".

Henar is lucky to come from an open-minded family, for some Kurdish girls are (in Western terms) heavily restricted by their families. They are not allowed to go on school trips, stay out at night or have relationships. This normally results in leading secret lives. As a result, they have to be extremely careful. Unfortunately, if they are seen by someone from the community while they are with their boy-friend, they can get into serious trouble, sometimes even endangering their lives. Heshu Yunis was a seventeen-year-old girl who was murdered and mutilated by her father on October 12th 2002. Heshu arrived in the UK when she was only three years old, she grew up here and was very much a Londoner. She was dating a young Lebanese man and was found out by her father, who threatened to kill her if she carried on seeing him. She promised to stop but carried on seeing her boy-friend secretly, thinking her father would not find out. Eventually her father killed her. I tried very hard to interview some of Heshu's Kurdish friends who knew about her problems with her father, but the parents of the young girls did not give their consent. Heshu had told her friends, a week before she was killed, that although her father kept threatening to kill her she did not think he will do it. He loved her too much, she had told her friends. She was the only girl in her family with two brothers. She was too young and possibly did not grasp the seriousness of the danger she was putting herself into.

2.4. Conclusion

When arriving in the country of refuge, a number of issues impede the well-being and progress of refugee women. The combination of experienced loss, adaptational requirements and having to wait until her asylum claim is processed, make the person feel powerless. Seeking asylum entails losing her place in a society she used to fit in, where she knew her environment and was loved by the people around her, losing the meaningful relationships in her life and living through a great deal of fear and uncertainty. The person then ends up isolated in a strange country, where she does not speak the language and feels alienated and shocked by some of the values and codes of behavior. The uncertainties experienced throughout this stage can cause the person to feel futile and powerless. Migration also changes the roles of women within their families and communities: it puts more burdens on their shoulders. Espin (1996) expresses this very well when she says, "Immigrant women have several mountains on their back". Even when the initial stages of adaptation are finished, women may suffer in different ways, by experiencing a change of status within the family, having more responsibilities, and being under more pressures.

The experience of lack of power over one's environment, the inability to control the course of events and the future, are of great importance when we are dealing with refugee women. This is particularly so because, as women, they already experience power differentials within their families and intimate relationships: losing control over the environment further disempowers them. Becoming members of the refugee community in exile means becoming a member of a stigmatized group. In the last few years there has been a major campaign against refugees by the British media. Refugees have been pictured as manipulative individuals who are swamping the country's resources because the UK is a 'soft touch'. They have been associated with terrorism and crime, and generally many negative words have been used about them. All these factors contribute to the process of alienation and powerlessness of refugees which is reflected in their world-views as well as perceptions of themselves.

According to structuralism, power differential and oppression lie at the roots of problems that people have in living (Burstow, 1992, Ch.1). Thus the exercise of power through agency and freedom in pursuing one's goals are central to the human existence. Through tracing existential themes that have entered feminist thinking, Burstow (ibid.) says:

> .....our human existence is predicted on our ability to project meaning, to embark on projects, to create world. As subjects we are forever creating and re-creating world by making new choices and by ordering what is around us. This world creating ability and

the transcendence of self and other that is involved distinguishes us from objects and to a lesser extent from other species.

In this sense, the frustration that refugee women experience in virtue of their gender and their living in situations which are out of their control, and hence losing some of their ability to embark on projects and create a world for themselves, leads to feelings of alienation, inadequacy and hopelessness, all of which feature in depression. The way to help this group of women should take into account the process which makes them powerless and try to reverse it by empowering them. Nevertheless, exile is not a completely negative experience. The participants of this research have spoken about freedom and opportunities previously not experienced by them. Women can be empowered by talking about their experiences (narrative therapy), by forming women's groups to deal with their needs and fight oppression, and by taking advantage of the opportunities which exile may have opened up for them. In the next section I will discuss each of these in turn.

3. EMPOWERMENT OF REFUGEE WOMEN

3.1. Narrative therapy as a form of empowerment

According to Weber (1998), race, class, gender and sexuality are socially constructed power relationships that empower one group and oppress another. In this sense, being white is privileged while being non-white is not. Being a man is privileged and being a woman is not. These categories, however, are deeply embedded in our everyday lives. Each of these categories, though socially constructed, are portrayed as linked to biology, implying that they are not changeable. This is why narrative therapy is important. The method takes into account the social construction of the self and reality. It is also relevant to refugee women because by virtue of their gender and their ethnicity (non-white and non-European) they are oppressed twice.

Swan (1998) provides an example which illustrates the social construction of some of our daily categories. When a child catches cold, Swan points out, there can be many reasons for this: onset of winter, tiredness, chance. However, the story that may dominate for the mother is that of her negligence. This is not accidental, but is constructed in her lived experiences within her community: the mother as nurturer, taking absolute care of her children, foreseeing problems and preventing them, and making sure that nothing goes wrong. In this sense if a woman fails to live up to society's expectations of her as a mother, she feels guilty and in doing so rules out other meanings and interpretations of the situation. Narrative therapy helps in revealing other possible interpretations and also in revealing the social construction of these expectations and who they serve, as opposed to seeing them as unchangeable rules of nature. It also helps women in highlighting the positive stories of survival and agency that have been overshadowed by internalized negative interpretations of themselves.

Herbst (1992) stresses the importance of empowerment and a holistic approach to health. She used the oral history method as a treatment for a group of Cambodian women refugees suffering from PTSD. These women had fled the Pol Pot regime and had lived in Thai camps for an average of four years before settling in the US. Living under a dictatorship and subsequently becoming refugees meant that they had lost power over the environment for a long period. They had many memory and attention problems which prevented them from learning English. Working for a minimal salary, they had ended up in high crime neighborhoods in Chicago, where they experienced racial prejudice and felt further disempowered. Herbst reports that through telling their stories, the women felt empowered and in control. The oral history gives positive meaning to their experiences as well as bringing them together into a support network. Through this method, trust, acceptance, release of anger and the re-forming of a supportive network developed. Herbst (1992) points out that asking them for their histories implies that trauma is only part of their experience. It stresses that the survivors are more than victims: "they are strong, they have survived". She quotes Kowalenko (1988, p.2):

> ......language externalizes as nothing else can. Thus oral history provides a picture, not a mere report of the experience but the experience itself. It represents human experiences as it has been or is being lived. When, during therapy, stories are told, data from the individual's life are retrieved and pressures are relieved thereby increasing self control.

Herbst also points out that the individual's self-esteem is also enhanced by the therapist's attitude to their attention, memory problems and somatic symptoms: "these are normal reactions to abnormal situations, it is not your fault". The therapist's respect for and interest in their histories further enhances their self-esteem. As the women hear stories similar to their own, the mutual display of feelings and support also re-establishes a sense of community. Postero (1992), also points out the importance of providing a safe environment and gradually establishing trust for refugees to be able to reveal and overcome the painful experiences they have survived.

Through my work as a writer with a group of refugee women in Essex I have found that women feel in control and empowered when they talk or write about their lives. The writing workshops initially were commissioned to make these women feel more positive about where they live: the project was called *A different light*. Yet despite reading their poems and encouraging them to think about where they live and the positive aspects of their new homes, most of the women preferred writing about their own countries and their former lives. The majority of the women were from Afghanistan, but there were also some Kurdish and Albanian women. For most of them, it was the first time they had ever tried to write and telling their own story: the story of their homeland made them feel that they are doing something useful.

At the performance held at the end of the project, each of the women had to choose one poem to read. Most of them chose poems about their homes and their lives. One of the Afghan women said to me: "I want people to know how wonderful Afghanistan was before the war, I want them to stop thinking of us as fundamentalists and backward". In her piece she concentrated on her youth, when women used to work and people dressed as they pleased. Writing in this way and then reading their work to the group also gave this group of women an opportunity to listen to each other's work and thus to create a support network. Through the group, the participants gradually started opening up to me and telling me more about their lives and current problems. Sometimes seeking my advice or asking me to interpret things for them. There was growing intimacy and some laughter about life and incidents from the past.

I shall quote a poem here by **Farzana**, an Afghan woman in her late twenties:

> In this country people are honest
> but in our country people are hospitable.
> We love and respect our parents very much
> and we never feel lonely
> but we are lonely here.
> Even English people are lonely here
> they live with their pets.

Espin (1992), speaking of her own personal experiences, says that she found that sharing her experiences producing a cathartic effect. In my own research I have also found that despite some tearful moments, especially when talking about the death of family members at home while they were absent, the participants felt resilient most of the time. This is partly because telling one's story to an interested audience gives us a sense of importance and satisfaction. It also helps us realize and understand the complex situations we may be facing. This realization in itself explains the anger or sadness we may feel about our situation and helps us realize that what we feel is in some way rational and justified. Most refugee stories are survivor stories. By talking about the difficulties they have faced and the things they have achieved, some of the women came to see themselves more as survivors and less as victims.

In this sense telling one's story helps the person understand her situation, come to terms with it, and draw from her inner strength and history in order to adjust and construct a more positive image of herself. It reminds the person how she has coped in the past and this can be empowering. Having said this, narrative therapy does not work for everyone. There are indeed women who prefer to not talk about certain things. I have spoken to many refugee workers during my research and some of them have pointed out to me that some women would rather chat, while others simply come for massage therapy. It is therefore useful to remember that although narrative therapy can be very useful to some women, it does not work for all of them.

3.2. Activism and women's groups as forms of empowerment

Women's groups are important because of the supportive environment they create when they can utilize their strength to fight oppression together. Light (1992) reports the activities of a group of Guatemalan refugee women in a camp in South Mexico. This organized group dealt with women's subordination without cutting ties with the home culture. According to Light, this is mainly because although the group deals with women's subordination, they identify traditional culture as progressive rather than oppressive. For this group of displaced women, traditional culture plays a unifying role and they use this as a framework to bring about change. Another important reason for not cutting ties with traditional culture is because of their belief in the main values of co-operation, the primacy of the community over the individual, and a strong connection to the natural world.

Women's groups can function as a support network or take on more political aims. The women's group I worked with in Essex mainly functioned as a support network. By providing a safe space where women can get together, they naturally bond and help each other by talking and sharing their lives. They benefit from the therapeutic effects of telling one's story as described in the previous section. Other groups, however, may have more political aims and aspire to bring about change for women of the community and back in the home country.

There are many Kurdish women's organizations in Britain. One of these is KWAHK, Kurdish Women Against Honor Killing. This group has managed to utilize the energy and inputs of a group of women to expose, condemn and combat violence and discrimination experienced by Kurdish women, both in the Diaspora and their homeland. KWAHK has played a great role in publicizing cases of violence against Kurdish women nationally and internationally. Representatives of the group have presented papers at conferences held in New York, Washington, London and Sweden, organized by high-profile international organizations (see www.kwahk.org). KWAHK also held the first Kurdish Women's conference on violence and honor killing in Paris, February 2002. It has also helped women's groups in Iraqi Kurdistan to put pressure on the Kurdish Regional Authorities, in order to change articles of the Iraqi penal court regarding honor killing, which permit men to kill women for reasons of honor or otherwise. It was due to KWAHK's campaigns and pressure from within that the Kurdish Regional government declared these articles redundant in 2000 and 2001. A man in Iraqi Kurdistan cannot get away with killing a woman for reasons of adultery or dishonor, neither can he take a second wife unless his first wife agrees. The law regarding inheritance has also changed and now, in contrast to the past, men and women inherit everything equally.

Traditionally any issue involving women and honor was not to be spoken about. By including these concepts in its name, the group was already making progress in naming and talking about the issue. KWAHK was also very much involved in the case of Abdulla Yunis who killed his seventeen year old daughter, Heshu. The group was asked to write a report about honor killing and later became part of the working group created by Metropolitan Police for this case. Abdulla Yunis tried to obtain release on bail. His friends and comrades set out to raise £250,000 for this purpose. It was only due to KWHAK's opposition that bail did not go through. The founder and representative of the group, Dr Nazand Bagikhani, pointed out that if Mr Yunis was released on bail, he would leave the country and go back to Kurdistan, evading justice. Eventually, on September 29th 2003, he was given a life sentence. Although the group was content that justice had been done, they were not happy about the media coverage of the event. This portrayed Mr Yunis as a traditional Muslim and the reason for the murder as Heshu's dating a Christian man. In fact, far from being a traditional Muslim, Abdulla Yunis was known within the community as 'Khula the Communist', and Heshu's boy-friend was a Muslim. The group carried on campaigning against what they perceived to be misrepresentation and racism. Honor killing, though it exists in the Kurdish community, is not specific either to Kurds or Muslims. This is another issue which KWAHK tried to expose and talk about.

The founder of the group, Dr Begikhani, was awarded the Emma Humphrey Memorial Prize and has been short-listed for the Right of Livelihood Award in Sweden for her dedication and ongoing work against violence directed at women in Kurdish communities. Members of the group are currently researching with other women's groups in their homelands in order to document victims of violence. Acting together to bring about more egalitarian gender roles in the society is another way for women to become active agents in their lives, hence reclaiming power and fighting for women's rights to create democracy.

The above examples all stress the importance for healing of two notions: life history and participation in the rebuilding and shaping of new communities. Both of these are essential as forms of empowerment. They allow women to draw on their inner strength and to support each other by understanding and processing what has happened and accepting it, as well as working together to rebuild their shattered lives and communities. It is also important when dealing with refugee women to have understanding of their culture and their experiences, so that relevant help is provided which is culturally and individually relevant.

3.3. Empowerment by taking advantage of opportunities in the host country

Migration, despite the difficulties it brings, can open many doors to women. Women migrants can take advantage of education and employment opportunities that may have not been open to them in their home countries. Economic independence can lead to a greater independence in other spheres. It gives room to escape from some oppressive traditions and to experience more freedom. My own experience in the Kurdish community suggests that women integrate more than men. After overcoming the initial difficulties, they are very open to take advantage of new possibilities, to revise their cultural values or feel freer to express their views. Men find accepting new norms more difficult, partly because the old ways serve them better. According to Islam alcohol is forbidden to both men and women, but culturally it is acceptable for men to drink and not for women. Sex before marriage is also forbidden for both genders, but again it is only women who are expected to abide by this rule. In her study with Asian Indian families in America, Dasgupta (1998) points out that the maintenance of tradition and identity is placed on women's shoulders. This is possibly why women are more strictly monitored than men. The women who have taken part in this research reported many ways in which migration has given them opportunities. I shall talk about each of these in turn.

3.3.1. Employment and education

Many of the young women who took part in this research feel empowered by the fact that they have many choices open to them. In contrast to their home countries, where they would have to go to university in order to find employment, there are many other courses and trainings available in the UK that do not require going to university.

Henar spoke about the lack of work opportunities back home. She pointed out that although women were allowed to study, very often they could not study what they wanted. First of all because there were strict requirements in terms of getting the right grades to do certain degrees. Here, Henar points out, there are many alternative universities that may take you with lower grades. Secondly, certain professions were made difficult by the Iraqi government. For example if you wanted to teach, you would have to become a member of the Ba'ath party. People who refused to join the Ba'ath party ended up staying at home despite being qualified teachers. Henar also pointed out that through living in an open society men and women work and study together and there is a lot more contact between the sexes. This, according to Henar, is essential for young people's development:

> Back home girls don't have any confidence, we don't know much about people and their psychology. Young women don't get to learn how to react in complex social environments. Here, you get more confident and you handle things better and can be accounted responsible. I believe you can achieve many things here if you have time and if you want to, there are many opportunities.

Lana also said that back home 'we saw opportunities on TV' but here 'they are a reality'. She feels that there is no limit to what you can achieve as you can study whatever you like, take vocational and training courses and become financially independent. Lana also likes the fact that unlike back home where you could only work in the field of your study, here you can find work in a different field.

3.3.2. Biculturalism

Some of the women pointed out that living in the UK has given them the opportunity to choose between two different sets of values and become more confident in expressing what they felt.

Mani always felt inadequate back home. She felt as if she was exiled within her own family and society. She often felt 'like a stranger'. In her home country she constantly felt discriminated against as a woman. She felt a lot was wrong in society and took refuge in reading the works of Nawal Saadawi (an Egyptian feminist). Reading these books reassured her that she was not alone and certainly not abnormal, it confirmed to her that a lot was wrong in the community. Coming to Britain, Mani believes, has made her feel more confident and hence more comfortable in expressing her thoughts. She believes that "coming to a new country, learning a new language, getting to know a different people" has broadened her horizons. Through her studies (MA in European Union Law) and through having access to internet and a wider range of media, she learned a lot about democratic systems. Still, Mani points out, after coming to the UK, she only 'found peace again' when she made peace with her own community. She experienced racism for the first time where she was studying. Her teacher kept trying to undermine her and once even asked her before the class, "have you ever used a book called how to use your brain?" Mani experienced a lot of disappointment in her first three years and 'felt more Kurdish and Eastern' than ever before. Mani has managed to find good values in both cultures:

> I feel that there are certain things which are international; they have nothing to do with West or East. They are more related to humanity, I do feel more humanitarian because here there is more democracy and human rights, and some of these values are ignored where we come from. But the warmth and social connectedness of our community, the romanticism does not exist here. When you join these together you have a more human and more international experience.

Mani strongly believes that it was only because of support from her family and friends, the warmth and caring that helped her cope with the difficulties she experienced. If it wasn't for the support of her Kurdish friends and her sister, she believes she would not have managed:

> Although I disapprove of certain things in my culture, there are many things in it that I'm proud of. People like us are privileged, we have two cultures and we can pick the best values from both. I try to be selective.

3.3.3. Freedom

Women can benefit from the more liberal social environment they find themselves in. The West has been associated with greater gender dichotomy and more egalitarian gender roles. In this sense, western society itself is less male dominated and hence a better place for women compared to societies where patriarchy is still dominant. The young women who contributed to this research talked about the greater freedom they enjoyed because they lived in an environment where they were less restricted by gossip and sexism.

Lana, who is her late twenties, said that she liked 'this place' because no one is looking at her and she can come and go freely. She comes from an open-minded family and her parents were less strict than most Kurdish parents. Still, the out-side community restricted her movements. Lana pointed out that she can 'do shopping without being watched', dress as she likes, study and work without any-one censuring her behavior, without anyone talking about her and asking her questions:

> 'There are many differences for us as women.. The freedom you have here, what you are worth is not like back home.'

On the other hand Mani, who is in her mid-thirties, pointed out that although she enjoys more freedom in the UK, she tries very hard to maintain traditions when in contact with members of the community. This is mainly because she wants to go back to Kurdistan one day. She feels free with her friends, but out of fear and respect for more traditional members of the community, she avoids doing certain things in front of them. For example, among Kurdish people she does not drink alcohol and dresses more conservatively. She describes her own behavior as a 'necessary hypocrisy'. She still fears people's responses and does not like shock-ing them. Sometimes she feels like a coward, but her reservations come from a mixture of fear and respect. She believes this is like leaving the door open behind her back: she does not want to cut ties with the community.

Dila, who is in her early fifties, has never been married. Back home she wanted to live alone but was not allowed to. She had to live with her older sister who was also single. Dila mentioned how although she has suffered a great deal of depression as a result of not having a job and losing her status, she loves being 'in this country':

> I have come to be free in this country, to live alone and do as I want. It may be too late but still at least when I sit down I can say what I think and do as I please, back home I didn't even have the freedom to do that.

Back home many people felt sorry for her because she had chosen not to get married; others always watched her and her sister. She is by nature a very humorous person, but back home she had to be very careful - not out of fear for herself, but for her brothers. She loved her brothers and did not want people to badmouth them because of her. She now lives on her own and tends to her garden.

Her only wish is to find a job in the UK – then, she says, her happiness would be complete.

Sheila, *who is from a less educated background, pointed out that gossip and bad-mouthing did not just affect women but also victimized men. She pointed out how her life has changed for the better here. She can now go out with her husband arm in arm without people talking. She feels that her husband has relaxed much more since he has been here and he is much more supportive, as a result of which she is happier. Back home on a number of occasions when Sheila was going out with her husband, seeing people they knew made him change his behavior. For example, he did not want his friends to see him walking arm in arm with his wife, this was considered being a woman's man and being soft. Also he would never carry the children if he saw anyone he knew; carrying children is considered a woman's job. Now, Sheila pointed out, her husband sees that doing such things is not considered bad. Because of the social setting, he is much more relaxed and helps her around much more than he used to.*

Two of the women participants of my research have also been able to escape abusive marriages while living in the UK. Both of them believe that they would have found it much more difficult if they were back home. Mainly because divorce is socially undesirable and most families put great pressure on their children never to consider divorce. It is also difficult particularly for women because divorced women are perceived with suspicion by the community, they are considered guilty. It is therefore more difficult to start a new life after divorce by finding another husband or living alone. Most divorced women end up living with their married brothers or sisters and live a restricted life.

Layla had been in a bad marriage back home for many years. When she came here with her young children she found her husband worse than he had been back home, having an affair, lying to her and hiding many things. Although he had never been a good husband, he was not physically abusive – but when she arrived in the UK and confronted him with his affair, he started beating her. Once he kicked her in the stomach so many times that although her period was not due, she started bleeding. She had tried to get divorced in Iraq but had not gone through with it because of her young children and the fact that her father was in the Kurdish opposition. She was worried that her husband would blackmail her about her father. Finally, when she arrived in the UK, she felt no more fear of the government or people's gossip. She decided to leave him. Fortunately she had been an English teacher back home and spoke fluent English. This helped her find a lawyer and file for a divorce without being scared:

> I told him that there was one strand of hair keeping us together and I had kept that connection because of our children, if anything goes wrong that connection will be lost forever. He said I was a coward, I would never be able to do such thing. I said okay I will prove to him how cowardly I am.

Leena *got married very young. She married her husband and came to the UK, totally isolated from anyone she knew. Soon she realized her husband had an incontrollable temper, but she kept hoping that he would change. Over the years he started beating her more and more. Nevertheless, she stayed with him for six years. Once she was six* *months pregnant and he beat her so badly that she had a miscarriage. He kept saying to her that she would never escape from him, he would cut her to pieces and throw the pieces in the river. She was too terrified to do anything. It was only when members of her family came over that she started confiding in them and telling them the truth. With support from her brothers she managed to leave him:*

> When I got divorced I felt as if I had just opened the door of the prison and escaped. For years I felt like I'm imprisoned for life, that I have no hope of escaping. I kept crying and thinking that's it, I will never be free again. Then when I got divorced I felt as if I had escaped this prison which I thought was for life. I ran away and my life started again, as if I was born again. At first of course I had no direction; I felt like a child who's recently walking and can't walk properly, I was so happy.

4. CONCLUSION

Refugee women experience great obstacles when they arrive in the host country. Dealing with loss as well as having to adapt to the new country in the absence of support network is greatly exhausting and very difficult. Many of the women I have interviewed reported being depressed at the earlier stages of their resettlement. Most refugees feel powerless facing the great bureaucratic system in Britain as well as having to wait and trying to learn. All these factors are interlinked. Women can be empowered by telling their stories, by forming women's groups to fight oppression and by taking advantage of the opportunities that are open to them. Integration and adaptation, however, are not without risk. Some young women who integrate and adopt more western values may face great resistance from their families and communities. Sometimes they may lose their lives because of the changes they undergo. Living between the sexism of their own community and racism of the outside community leaves them experiencing great anxieties and pressures. They have to be very careful if they are to survive this process, they have to keep negotiating their two worlds.

REFERENCES

Burstow, B. (1992) *Radical Feminist Therapy: Working in the context of violence.* London: Sage Publications.

Dasgupta, S.D. (1998) Gender roles and cultural continuity in the Asian Indian immigrant community in the US. *Sex Roles 38*, 953-655.

Espin, O. M. (1992) Roots uprooted: the psychological impact of historical/ political dislocation. In E. Cole, O. M. Espin, and E. D. Rothblum (eds.), *Refugee women and their mental health: shattered societies, shattered lives.* New York, London & Norwood: Harrington Park Press.

Espin, O. M. (1996) 'Race', racism, and sexuality in the life narratives of immigrant women. In Wilkinson, S. (ed.), *Feminist Social Psychologies: International Perspectives.* Scarborough: Open University Press, 87-103.

Herbst, (1992) From helpless victim to empowered survivor: oral history as a treatment for survivors of torture. In E. Cole, O. M. Espin, and E. D. Rothblum (eds.), *Refugee women and their mental health: shattered societies, shattered lives.* New York, London & Norwood: Harrington Park Press.

Light, D. (1992) Healing their wounds: Guatemalan refugee women as political activists. In E. Cole, O. M. Espin, and E. D. Rothblum (eds.), *Refugee women and their mental health: shattered societies, shattered lives.* New York, London & Norwood: Harrington Park Press.

Postero (1992) On trial on the promised land: seeking asylum. In E. Cole, O. M. Espin, and E. D. Rothblum (eds.), *Refugee women and their mental health: shattered societies, shattered lives.* New York, London & Norwood: Harrington Park Press.

Swan, V. (1998) Narrative therapy, feminism, and race. In Seu, I. B. & Heenan, C. M. (eds.), *Feminism and psychotherapy: Reflections on contemporary theories and practices.* London, Thousand Oaks, New Delhi: Sage Publications, 30-42

Weber, L. (1998) A conceptual framework for understanding race, class, gender and sexuality. *Psychology of Women Quarterly 22*,13-32

10. BEYOND THE PERSONAL PAIN:
Integrating social and political concerns in therapy with refugees

Julia Bala[1]

1. RE-STARTING A MEANINGFUL LIFE

"I still have my life" said Dima (an unaccompanied adolescent from Africa) quietly, after a long break that followed the seemingly endless list of her losses and painful experiences. Her short sentence reflected a deep sadness for everything she had lost, but it also signaled a triumph of the survivor ready to pick up the threads of her life and go on. Like many refugees, Dima is confronted not only with the painful experiences of the past, but also with many open questions: How to make sense of what has happened? How to reorganize life in the unfamiliar new world? How to re-dream the future? The refugee experience can be seen as a cycle of disruptions, losses and transitions, where the central question that each refugee has to face is: how to re-start a meaningful life? Or, as K. Abdullah, an Iranian writer living in the Netherlands put it: a refugee needs to find out how to unravel anew the riddle of life.

Refugees arriving in Europe are confronted with the almost impossible task of making peace with the past while faced with a lengthy asylum procedure with uncertain outcome, of re-establishing the disrupted stability and continuity within an unstable, unpredictable situation. They have to regain control over their lives while being in a position of powerlessness, to re-stage a future life while the perspectives seem to be closed. Mental health professionals working to assist refugees are confronted with similar questions, dilemmas and paradoxes. Many theories, methods and techniques have been developed in the last few decades from which mental health professionals can choose their approach to the complex problems of refugees. Different approaches emphasize different aspects (medical-psychological, psychosocial or cultural) of the refugee experience. Whatever choice is made, it is essential that we never lose sight of the fact that the task for refugees is to solve an existential riddle and find a way to live a meaningful life despite what has happened to them, in the face of extremely difficult conditions in the present and an often still uncertain future.

---

[1] Julia Bala, Centrum '45, De Vonk, Amsterdam, The Netherlands.

1.1. Focusing the therapeutic lenses

The mental health provider confronted with the complex problems of refugees faces certain questions and dilemmas: should one see the refugees as survivors, as victims, as medical causalities, as traumatized people or as marginalized citizens? Should one reduce the problems in order to make them manageable, or should one expand the context to understand problems in their complexity? Where are the problems located: within the individual, the family and the community, or within the interactions among different system levels? Should the problems be defined as psychological, medical, social, political, cultural, existential or multidimensional? One can choose to transcend the either/or attitude and search for a broad conceptual frame.

Whenever a child or an adolescent is referred to treatment, he or she brings into the treatment room the family members – those who are here, those who were left behind, those who are missed and/or no longer alive. From fragments of memories of a past violent reality in the country of origin and fragments of the troublesome current life-world, each family tries to construct a narrative, to make sense of the experience.

Luria, a pale, silent, withdrawn 15-year-old from the Middle East, overwhelmed with anxieties and hopelessness, can not concentrate any longer in school. Since the family's asylum request had been refused for a second time, he is preoccupied with the increasing threat of being sent back to the country of origin and his future perspectives became closed. Confronted with the insecure future, Luria gave up his attempts to anchor himself in the present. He does not want to go to school any more. Even when, under pressure from his parents, he does go to school, he stays in the corridors instead of joining the class. Learning or being with peers does not make sense any longer. The surplus of past and present problems that he is struggling with, or those he projects into the future – none of this he can share with his peers. He feels even more lonely in presence of his classmates, whose reality he experiences as so different from his own. At home, in a small room of the asylum center, he feels unhappy as the tensions and conflicts among the family members mount. Luria is overwhelmed with worries about the future, scared that the increasing conflicts between his father and mother might end in a divorce, leading to the last fragmentation of the already separated family.

His father does not respond immediately to the questions addressed to him. His words emerge slowly, as if each word uttered is painful. What should he say? He told his story too many times. He lost his hope long time ago. There is nothing to be said, expected or done. Did the father lose his hope after his village was destroyed, or while witnessing extreme forms of human violence? Perhaps the hope slipped away during the long years of hiding or during the imprisonment, or when the family finally arrived to a safe place but the authorities distrusted their accounts of the past. Perhaps the hope eroded further later, during the five years of uncertainty about the asylum procedure. At night, Luria's father is pursued by the intruding memories of the past. During the day he sits in the tiny one-room apartment, overwhelmed with threatening thoughts about an uncertain future. Luria's father believes he has failed: as a professional, as a political activist, as a father and as a husband. He experiences himself as a ruined man.

His mother tries to be strong and stay in control. Only the deep dark circles under her eyes betray her worries: about her husband, once a man of influence, who became powerless; about her successful son facing defeat; about the weakening of the family ties under the pressure of ongoing threats. Luria's mother tries to keep the years spent under threat, the longing for family members who were left behind, the sadness for her lost brother, far away. It seems that only the memories of some quiet moments in their previous life, the lack of hope for the future and the overwhelming anxieties remain as the glue holding this family together. Luria's mother tries with her remaining strength to hold the weakened family together and to keep going, despite her deep despair.

The intertwined problems of refugee families appear often as a difficult puzzle: in which way did the armed conflicts, political oppression and the forced migration disrupt the life course of a child and his family? In which way did the violence, the losses, the uncertain outcome of the asylum procedure, change the relations and roles of family members? How did the accumulated stressful events shatter the beliefs and assumptions of Luria, his father and mother, and how have these changes altered their expectations, mutual relations and their relatedness to the outside world? The unpredictable length and outcome of the asylum procedure, the insecure future, erase goals, reduce expectations and makes anchoring in the present impossible.

1.2. Kaleidoscope instead of prism: a developmental-systemic perspective

The mental health professional needs integrated, kaleidoscopic conceptual lenses that are broad and adjustable enough to allow the understanding of the complex problems and cultural diversities of the refugees. Exploring the interplay of internal (biological, psychological) and external (familiar/cultural/social/political) influences that hinder or facilitate development through various system levels, as described by Ciccheti and Cohen (1995), helps to evaluate the risk factors and protective factors in both the developmental and the socio-environmental context. Identifying the threats posed by social and political changes, altered family relations, beliefs and expectations, helps to map the influences that interfere with the fulfillment of developmental tasks.

Van der Veer (1997) distinguishes three developmental interferences in the lives of refugees: the primary developmental interference, prior to the political changes that led to organized violence, the secondary developmental interference linked to traumatization caused by political factors, and the tertiary occurring after the flight, connected to painful experiences endured in the country of exile. In which way did traumatization and uprooting interfere with the development of individual family members and of the family as a whole? In which way did the lengthy hiding and separation affect the relations between Luria's father and mother, in which way did the years spent in jail change his father's assumptions about the world, and how did the changes in his relations and assumptions affect the development of Luria? How did the hung asylum procedure, the lack of recognition and safety, affect the family's beliefs and interactions? In the same way it is essential to understand the individual, family, community and socio-cultural factors and processes that facilitate the adaptation of family members, that help them to cope with series of misfortunes and which help them to re-establish their disrupted life course.

The consequences of stressful experiences can be seen as individual problems, but also as family problems and problems within the broader system levels. Even when only one family member is traumatized or develops acute stress reactions, all family members become affected. When more family members struggle with the consequences of cumulative stress, further distress is created by dysfunctional interactions that undermine mutual support in the family. The appraisal of the individual within the family, and the family within the past and current socio-political and cultural context, includes "global trends in policy, politics and philosophy, through more local, social and cultural processes to personal coping" (Ager, 2000). Basic information about the political situation that forced refugees to flight, the political situation in the country of arrival, attitudes and policies that influence the life conditions and rights of asylum seekers and refugees, creates a context for understanding the life world of the refugees.

Family members share different interpretations of the past and current events that affect their lives. Their efforts to make sense of the experience are influenced not only by personal and family beliefs and assumptions, but also by broader socio-political and cultural ideologies and discourses. Whether one is seen as a hero or a traitor in the country of origin, a recognized refugee or an intruder in the country of arrival, influences how refugees define themselves, the others and the world. The mental health professional needs to explore the interaction between the internal and external meaning systems and understand how "the dominant beliefs in culture color the nature of experiences in families" and shape the actions, feelings and interpretations of the refugees (Dallos, 1997). Treatment requires a combination of individual, family and community interventions, interventions that include the 'significant system' (Boscolo and Bertrando, 1993) embracing those connected to the problem. The significant system of a refugee can be narrow or broad, but "the question is not how many people are in the room, but how many are in the therapist's head" (Haley, 1981).

2.   APPROACHING PROBLEMS IN THEIR COMPLEXITY

2.1. The Cumulative Effect of the Stressors

The interplay of disruptive processes of traumatization, uprooting and marginalization affects children and families differently, according to the developmental stage and the stage of the family life cycle. In the experience of refugees the consequences of stressful events can be intertwined in many ways. Searching for the synergetic effect of the stressors means understanding the joint consequences of different events and the meaning of one event in the context of the other.

The door opens suddenly, in the same violent way as it was opened when the solder entered the house in an African village and attacked Jori's mother many years ago. It is the same door that appears in the 14-year-old boy's recurrent nightmares, , through which the police enter his apartment in the Netherlands, to take him by force to the airport and deport him back to the country of origin.

The scene has partially changed in the dream, but the intensity of the threat and the anxieties he experiences are the same. The painful past does not just simply slip into the future in a form of traumatic expectation; the anxieties are not just projected in the future, but are fortified by a new realistic threat – of being deported and sent back into the unsafe world. The traumatic past and the anticipated future threat are intertwined in the dream of Jori, as they are often intertwined in the daily life of the refugees. Is it a painful past that interferes with the commitment to the present for Luria's parents, or do family members have difficulties "making peace with the past" (Figley, 1989) because they are too busy coping with the ongoing anxieties and worries triggered by the long lasting insecurity? Is the mourning process in the family blocked by the traumatic experiences or by current stress? Or is the mourning process temporarily dissociated to facilitate the process of coping and adaptation of family members?

These are some of the tasks that refugee families face: to make peace with the past, to re-organize the relations within the fragmented family, to redefine the roles and rela- tions within the changed family structure, to adjust to a new environment and to reset the future perspectives. Each of these tasks opens for family members many questions and dilemma's: to talk or not to talk about the painful events in the past, what to forget and what to remember, how to explain what has happened, which norms and values to keep, which ones to alter? Family members need to redistribute the roles and tasks that previously belonged to the members of the extended family, to define in which way to stay in contact with those who are left behind, and what sort of new contacts to build up (and with whom). Traumatization, prolonged grief or chronic distress interfere with stabilization and the adjustment of the family members to the new environment, and sometimes undermine severely parents' efforts to meet children's' needs. Certain fixed, long-lasting dysfunctional patterns of adjustment built around life adversities can create more risk for the future functioning of family members than the traumatic event itself. The intertwined problems appear sometimes as an entangled yarn of wool (Van Essen, Somers and Bala, 1996). Finding the right thread to unravel it means setting the priorities jointly with family members and defining the starting point of the treatment.

2.2. Prioritizing change

When the accumulated stressful events are intertwined, it is preferable to map prior- ity areas of change as described by Hanna & Brown (1995): by defining the problem that is of most immediate importance to the family, the problem that has the greatest negative consequence if not handled, the problem that can be corrected most easily, considering the resources and constraints, and the problem that requires handling before other problems can be solved. In Luria's family, the shared belief that the interminably bogged-down asylum procedure blocked their efforts to make peace with the past and re- start a new life aggravated their powerless position. Family members were mainly worried about the escalation of conflicts that would deprive them of mutual support. To introduce a minimum of stability in the family life, a combination of individual, family and community interventions seemed justified. Reducing the current stress and its impact often requires often practical aid, combined with symptom control and alteration of dysfunctional interactive patterns, aimed at stabilizing the family unit as a necessary precondition for creating space for the integration of fragmented experiences form the past and re-opening future perspectives (Bala, 2001; Van Essen, 1999).

2. 3. The synergetic interplay of protective factors and processes

An interesting question is whether the protective processes also have a synergetic, cumulative effect. Resilient children have a mixture of personal resources (sense of mastery, social skills, high self-esteem), together with social support from parents, teachers or the larger community (Gore and Eckenrode, 1996). The protective factors seems to work together, influencing each other through various processes: for instance, social support has the effect of increasing self-esteem, shaping realistic appraisals of the situation and one's ability to cope with it, and increasing coping options (Robinson and Garber, 1995). Exploring not only what is lost but also what remains, not only the source of vulnerabilities but also the sources of protection and resilience, is the first step towards empowering refugees.

Discovering how family members tried to cope with the stressful events, what they found helpful up to now, how they support each other and what sort of external support they find acceptable, means mapping the domains of the hidden strength of each family member and the family as a whole. If the assumption is that protective factors and coping efforts are interconnected and have a synergetic effect, introducing minimal changes such as emphasizing positive statements, interactions, behavior (Hanna & Brown, 1995), facilitating open communication and mutual support, broadening the coping repertoire of family members, would reinforce the functional adaptation of family members and of the family as a whole. The assumption that "resilience can be forged even when problems cannot be solved" (Walsh, 1998) is essential in working with refugee families, especially when some of the factors that create the problems cannot be immediately influenced. The adolescent who concludes that he still has many problems but knows better how to deal with them, has more chance to face not only the stressors originating from the past and present, but also those that he needs to face in the future.

3. THE NEXUS OF PERSONAL AND POLITICAL DIMENSIONS OF THE PROBLEMS

Should mental health professionals focus their attention on social and political factors or the personal, inner representational lives of refugees? Mental health providers aware of the possible traps often face dilemma's: how much does our political understanding lead to excessive focus on the external facts, at the cost of the inner and relational *representations* of the external facts? Or to put it the other way around: how can we understand socially caused problems from a purely constructivist point of view (Walter & Adam, 2000) Refugees themselves are often faced with this puzzle and try to find different ways of approaching it. *In which way have the political events shaped my intimate life?* is the focal question around which H. B., a Holocaust survivor and a former refugee, tries to shape his memories into a book. From a calm distance, he explores the dynamic of relations between external and internal, between political and personal, between collective and individual history. B.'s approach shapes a viable paradigm where the problems are located in neither the political nor the personal domain, but in their nexus.

Mental health professionals generally attach more value to individual than to structural (social, cultural, political) factors and tend to use internalizing explanations of the problems, while refugees more often connect their problems to the structural factors (Kramer, 1999; see Chapter 8). Refugees expect mental health professionals to show more understanding of their social and political aspects of their lives. Some therapists, such as Van der Veer (1992/1998) also find this important, suggesting that the political aspects of the problems need to be addressed and recognized, even when problems cannot be solved. There are also refugees that tend to internalize problems instead of experiencing the problems as consequences of external events, seeing themselves as being a problem instead of experiencing themselves in relation to a problem as described by Weingarten (1998), Dallos, (1997). Family members may be overwhelmed by inten-sive guilt feelings or mutual blame, overlooking the broader social political events that influenced their lives. The father of Farid turns his days and nights into self-torture, accusing himself for not being able to secure his family refugee status. Family members blame him for his late decision to leave the country and ascribe the physical injury of his 14-years-old son to him. The external forces leading to both events are left out of account by family members. Engaging in clinical reflection on the way in which oppressive ideologies and practices might be influencing family members is, according to Dallos (1997), a valid component of therapy. Locating the origins of events in the domain where they belong helps to differentiate the personal and political domains and to understand their interplay. Mental health professionals should not be locked into the individual meanings of events, nor should they become fixated on political processes and collective meanings. Instead, they should help refugees to search for the inter-connectedness of political events and personal meanings and in which way these inter-locked processes affect their lives.

3.1. Between the private and the public domain

The testimony method, developed in Chile during the 1970's, became one of the approaches that attempt to integrate the private pain with the political context. When political refugees give testimony about the torture to which they have been subjected, the trauma story can be given a meaning, can be reshaped: private pain can be transformed into political dignity (Agger & Jensen, 1990).

In one of the recent applications of the testimony method, the narrative of the shock-ing events is recorded, typed by the therapist, read aloud and signed by the victim of organized violence as well as the therapist. Refugees receiving a copy of their testimony can for example decide whether to keep it, send it to a human rights organization, use it for the juridical process (Van Dijk & Schreuder, 2001), or leave a copy for the Oral History Archive of the Project on genocide, psychiatry and witnessing (Weine, 2001). The testimony method covers both the private and the public domain, and according to Weine it moves the trauma story outside the narrowing prisms of individual psycho-pathology and the psychotherapeutic dyad. It reframes the survivor's story in the social and historical context where the etiologic factor of state-sponsored violence originally took place. Even though the testimony method has a limited applicability (Van Dijk & Schreuder, op. cit.; Van der Veer, 1992/1998; Weine, op. cit.), the tendency to move a step beyond the personal pain by including the political and historical dimensions of the events takes us a step beyond than the private domain of the problems.

Even when the testimony method is not one of the chosen approaches of the mental health provider, refugees need to get information whenever possible about the options for de-privatizing their pain outside the therapy room – for example, by giving evidence about the political repression, torture and violence to human rights organizations and other for a such as war tribunals. The statement that "some refugees need treatment, but all need social justice" (Summerfield, 1999) can serve as a reminder for mental care professionals that clients need to have opportunities outside the therapy room, whether they choose to use them or not.

4. SOCIAL AND POLITICAL ASPECTS OF REFUGEE PROBLEMS IN THE POST-MIGRATION PERIOD

How asylum seekers are received in a country, which policies are followed concerning asylum procedure, reception or family reunion, depends on the current political and economic situation in the country, the predominating attitude toward asylum seekers, the possible access to a community network, and the availability of non-professional and professional help (medical, juridical, social).

Many refugees connect their psychological problems to the political and social aspects of their lives in the country of reception, rather than to the experiences in their country of origin (Boomstra & Kramer, 1997; Sveaass & Reichelt, 2001). In the first phase of their arrival in the host country, refuges are extremely vulnerable when confronted with several factors that are either stressful themselves, or limit their capacities to cope with the consequences of previous painful experiences. The long-drawn-out asylum procedure without a certain outcome, the lack of privacy, forced passivity in the reception centers, humiliation and discrimination, are experienced as extremely stressful and interfere with the attempts of refugees to cope with the past painful experiences and adjust to the recipient country. The uncertainty makes it difficult for asylum seekers to re-establish a feeling of security, predictability, role identity and commitment to the present: it aggravates existing psychological problems and triggers new ones.

The psychological consequences of socio-political factors in the host country are defined and treated by mental health professionals in various ways. They can be:-

a) denied, e.g. defined as attempts by the refugees to externalize their problems;
b) recognized, but defined as belonging outside the domain of professional expertise;
c) recognized, but seen as contra-indications for therapy (the asylum procedure undermines the security necessary for treatment);
d) seen as relevant, but secondary to traumatic experiences;
e) recognized as stressors that can lead new psychological problems or aggravate existing ones.

The mental health professional needs to explore and deal with the consequences of current socio-political factors as carefully as he or she does with complaints originating in the past, in order to understand their meaning and the consequences they have for refugees lives. The meaning of the current situation' – which is characterized in some European countries by lengthy waits in asylum centers, with a concomitant lack of privacy, work and possibilities for meaningful activities – needs to be understood in its connection to the past experiences of the refugees and the future perspectives. The resulting feelings of helplessness and frustration are compounded by pre-existing post-traumatic symptoms and unresolved grief. Some refugees experience their stay in asylum center as a second phase of powerlessness and isolation. Others believe that the restricted living conditions and the uncertain future, or the lack of privacy or social involvement, prevents their recovery from past experiences. Refugees spending years in an asylum center separated from their families are overwhelmed with guilt feelings, feelings of powerlessness, and apathy. Those who have already received a negative decision and are still in appeal, struggle with a blocked present and an inability to generate future perspectives, and are often overwhelmed with anxieties about the possibility of deportation. Being forced to leave the country of origin and not being yet accepted, means that there is no place for one in the world.

Through the years spent in an unsafe environment, not being able to visit even the most nearby shops, 12-year-old Tanja learned after a violent attack on her parents that they had to leave because there was no place for them in their own country. After their asylum request was refused, she learned that there is also no place for them here. Where to belong? At night Tanja stays awake, alert for sounds and shadows: is it the shadow of one of the refugees acting in despair, breaking the windows, like last week, or the steps of a policemen coming to deport them?

The resemblances with past situations became a trigger for traumatic experiences, aggravate them or are experienced as a repetitive cycle of disempowering experience. When the present situation is filtered through painful past experiences, when an asylum center is seen as a sort of concentration camp, the past and the present situation, the internal and external experiences need to be carefully differentiated and separated from each other (Van Essen, 2000). The mental health professional can assist in reducing the impact of the current stresses, widening the coping alternatives and taking practical actions when necessary to help improve the developmental context of refugee children and families, in effect becoming a mediator between the refugees and asylum center, lawyers and Ministry of Justice (Drozdek, 1998).

4.1. Between Engagement and Neutrality

The psychological symptoms tend to decrease for refugees who are granted a residence permit, as the time passes after resettlement (Silove, 2000). However, the interplay of old and new stressors can sometimes overshadow the lives of many refugees even after they are settled. Worries about missing family members or those perhaps still in mortal life danger, and prolonged separation form family members, can be accompanied by social isolation, unemployment, marginalized status and practical problems, which all have a special meaning in an unfamiliar environment. Risk is transformed into psychopathology through an accumulation of day-to-day tensions and adverse life changes in the absence of protective factors (Cohler et al., 1995). A situational analysis (Van der Veer, 1992/1998) needs to include the context of the present problems and the meanings refugees attach to it. What meaning the therapist is giving to these situations is also relevant. Would the therapist define them as external situational difficulties that should stay outside the mental health professional's concerns, or as additional stressors that interfere with the functional adjustment of family members?

Practical aid aimed at reducing risks that can lead to mental health problems or aggravate them, can be considered as justified preventive or therapeutic interventions. Connecting family members with other members of the interdisciplinary team or with formal organizations or informal groups that can offer informational and instrumental support around social and juridical issues, family reunion and tracing missing family members, is often the first step in supporting the stabilization of family members. Facilitating connections with the community network helps the refugees to validate the political, religious and other values and maintain the sense of continuity and self-esteem according to Richman (1998). Practical aid means, for example, opening up possibilities for utilizing the existing community resources, or reducing the cumulative stress that interferes with the functional adjustment of family members.

4.2. The Refugee Family in Cultural Transition

Acculturation is a process that includes not only changes in values, norms, beliefs and practices, but also changes in the social and political forces that have shaped the family life. Understanding the way in which cultural transitions affect the lives of family members requires a broad definition of culture to include age, gender, race, religion socio-economic status as well as the stage of migration. The therapist can support the adaptation to life in the recipient country only if he/she has respect for the cultural background of the refugees, recognizes their capacities and social status in the country of origin and has a critical distance to his/her own culture.

Conflicting cultural expectations and demands can be manifested within and among different system levels. Problems due to different beliefs, perceptions and practices can be created between family members and institutions, among family members having a different tempo of acculturation, or can be experienced as internalized identity conflicts. Even when the mental health provider has a good insight into the cultural background of the refugees, the cultural constructions of the family members need to be carefully explored, especially those that interfere with the adaptation. Which specific cultural demands are conflicting and interfering with the developmental tasks of the child or the family? Which relations in the family are threatened? How do differences between children and parents in the tempo of acculturation create problems? How do cultural definitions of race, gender and class create difficulties for family members? Operation-alizing the problems caused by different cultural perceptions and expectations as experienced by family members is the first step in making them manageable.

5. THE MENTAL HEALTH PROFESSIONAL IN THE SOCIETY

5.1. Co-creating realities

The interest of mental health professionals in the last two decades has been predominantly focused around the pathological dimensions of the refugee experience, with special attention being given to post-traumatic stress disorder. Historically, PTSD certainly played an important role in obtaining professional and public recognition of the long-lasting consequences of organized violence, and in opening up possibilities for refugees to get access to mental health care. But the increasing tendency to generalize the pathological and disempowering dimensions of the refugee experience in the professional and public discourse has also created some unfavorable side effects. A G. Stefanovski (2004) a Macedonian playwright described recently how patiently he tries to explain to people in UK, without success, that he is not a "bleeding-heart refugee" with PTSD. I wonder to what extent we – psychologists, psychotherapists and related professionals – are at least partially responsible for the tendency to see refugees as damaged people instead of messengers of human right violations, or people challenged to re-discover a meaningful life under extremely difficult conditions. Our theories, based on pathological processes, are becoming part of a reality constructed around refugees, leading sometimes to generalizations that all refugees are traumatized. In Sweden, Eastmond et al. (1994) have connected the increasing interest in psychological services for refugees with the lack of work opportunities for them, asking themselves whether this new focus might unwittingly set up and maintain sick roles in absence of other structures through which to reconstitute a meaningful life.

Perhaps the dominating disempowering images about refugees overshadow some-times the fact that the majority of refugees manage to make peace with the past and gradually find ways to re-start their disrupted life. The central question according to Summerfield (1997) is not so much how or why individuals became psychosocial causalities, but how or why the vast majority does not? Different factors and processes that facilitate adaptation and help re-starting a meaningful life, despite severe adversities, have been mapped, carefully described and classified years ago (Cichettli & Cohen, 1995; Rutter, 1987, 1996; Gore & Eckenrode 1996; McCubbin & McCubbin, 1989; Helmreich, 1992) but this literature remained for a long time on the margin of the interest of mental health professionals involved with refugees. The increasing tendency in the last decade to approach the refugee experience not only in terms of traumatic experiences and losses, but also in terms of strength and potentials for growth, creates possibilities for better understanding of the experience of the refugees, and also many alternatives for the mental health professional. Treatment approaches that emphasize the need for empowering refugees require more social engagement from professionals. Beside broadening up the coping strategies and strengthening the protective factors within the individual and the family, the mental health professional needs to understand the dynamic of community resources that influences the lives of the refugees.

5.2. From separating to mediating between private and public domain

In his article "The survivors syndrome: private problem and social repression", A. de Swaan (1982) describes how mental health providers created twenty years ago a buffer zone between the private and the public domain, concerning the problems of the concentration camp survivors. By being open to listening and to containing individual suffering, the mental health professionals were, according the author, protecting their clients against public indifference and lack of understanding. At the same time, mental health providers were protecting the community against the upsetting memories and emotions of the survivors. De Swaan's conclusion is that history cannot be worked through in consulting rooms alone: historical and political phenomena have to be worked through in the forum of public opinion. Twenty years later at a psychoanalytic conference in South Africa, R. Goldstone the former prosecutor of the International Tribunal for War Crimes in the former Yugoslavia, underlined the importance of public acknowledgement of the victim, and recognition by society. How can the recognition of the victim be acknowledged in society if it stays closed in the therapist room?

To what extent are we, as mental health care providers working with refugees, trapped in a similar process of buffering between refugees and society? What does our buffering function include? Is it only the pain of people who are victims of the atrocities of organized violence that stays, thanks to our 'containing', locked in the therapist room, or do we also contain and protect the community from the psychological consequences of the current policies for asylum seekers in the EU? In the public domain there is little awareness of the risks created by these policies for asylum seekers. By contrast, there is ample awareness of the threats and problems that refugees are supposed to create for the community. Do mental health professionals contribute, by helping some referred individuals, to the maintenance of ongoing risk to the psychological well-being of asylum seekers, and to blocking the process of making peace with the past, by not signaling the problems that are originating from the current asylum polices.?

Therapy can achieve limited goals, but it cannot eliminate the underlying societal forces that shape people's experiences (Dallos, 1997). Changing social realities is certainly not the primary task of therapist sitting face to face with the clients in the room. But the question is whether mental health professionals could contribute to changing certain policies that are blocking the process of recovery of refugees. Once outside the therapy room, mental health providers can point out links between individual problems and socio-political influences, can give scientific evidence on the risks that current reception practices create for refugees, and can suggest preventive measures that can reduce these risks and facilitate the successful adaptation of refugees. The role of the mental professional working with refugees extends beyond direct face-to-face contact, to *advocacy:* to efforts to create more optimal conditions for asylum seekers, and to enable them to organize themselves to help each other, as Van der Veer (1999) has suggested, instead of making them believe that they should either cope as individuals or seek professional help. By signaling the risks and strengthening community resources, the mental health professional would also manage to maintain the optimal neutrality in the therapy, and the optimal balance between the individual and societal without artificially dividing the private and public domain. Opening the door to dialogue with those *outside* the mental health professions – sociologists, anthropologists, politicians, human right activists, lawyers and journalists - can help to develop insight into the side-effects of the role of mental health workers. In this way therapy with refugees becomes a balancing act, between personal and socio-political domains, between private and public, between pain and empowerment.

REFERENCES

Ager, A. (2000) A constructivist framework for the analysis of children's response to organized violence. In: L. Van Willigen (ed.), *Heath Hazards of Organised Violence in Children II. Coping and Protective Factors*, 21-29. Utrecht: Stichting Pharos.

Agger I. & Jensen S.B. (1990) Testimony as Ritual and Evidence in Psychotherapy for Political Refugees. *Journal of Traumatic Stress 3*, 115-129.

Bala, J. (2001) Mother doesn't laugh any more. Therapeutic interventions with traumatized refugee families. In M. Verwey (ed.), *Trauma and Empowerment*. Berlin: VWB-Verlag.

Boscolo, L. & Bertrando, P. (1993) *The Times of Time. A New Perspective in Systemic Therapy and Consultation*. New York: W.W. Norton & Company.

Boomstra, R. & Kramer, S.A. (1997) *Cultuurverschillen in interacties tussen hulpverleners en vluchtelingen*. Utrecht: ISOR.

Carter, B. & McGoldrick M. (1989) *The Changing Family Life Cycle. A Framework for Family Therapy*. Boston: Allyn and Bacon.

Cicchetti, D. & D.J. Cohen. (1995) *Perspectives on Developmental Psychopathology*. In: D. Cicchetti & D.J. Cohen (eds.), *Developmental Psychopathology. Theory and Methods*, 3-23. New York: Wiley.

Cohler, B., Stott, F., & Musick, J. (1995) Adversity, vulnerability, and resilience: Cultural and developmental perspectives. In: D. Cicchetti & D.J. Cohen (eds.), *Developmental psychopathology. Theory and Methods*, 753-800. New York: Wiley.

Dallos, R. (1997) *Interacting Stories. Narratives, Family Beliefs and Therapy*. London: Karnac Books

Drozdek, B. (1998) Getraumatiseerde asielzoekers en vluchtelingen. *Maandblad Geestelijke Volksgezondheid 53*, 490-501.

Eastmond, M., Ralphsson, L. & Alinder, B. (1994) The Psychological Impact of Violence and War. Bosnian Refugee Families and Coping Strategies. *Refugee Participation Network 16*, 7-9.

Figley, C. R. (1989) *Helping Traumatized Families*. San Francisco: Jossey-Bass Publishers.

Gore S. & Eckenrode, J. (1996) Context and process on risk and resilience. In: Haggerty, R.J., Sherrod, L.R., Garmezy, N., Rutter, M. (eds.), *Stress, Risk and Resilience in Children and Adolescents*, 19-64. Cambridge: Cambridge University Press

Hanna, S.M. & Brown, J.H. (1995) *The Practice of Family Therapy. Key Elements Across Models*. Pacific Grove: Brooks/Cole Publishing Company.

Haley, J. (1981) *Reflections on Therapy*. Washington: The Family Therapy Institute.

Helmreich, W. B. (1992) *Against All Odds: holocaust survivors and the successful lives they made in America*. New Brunswick: Transaction Publishers.

Kramer, S.A. (1999) *Het psychologiseren van politieke ervaringen*. Utrecht: ISOR.

McCubbin, M.A. & McCubbin H.I. (1989) Theoretical orientations to family stress & coping. In: C.R. Figley (ed.), *Treating stress in families*, 3-45. New York: Brunner-Mazel.

Pynoos, R.S., Steinberg R. & Wraight R. (1995) A developmental model of childhood traumatic stress. In: D. Cicchetti & D.J. Cohen (eds.), *Developmental Psychopathology. Theory and Methods*, 72-96. New York: Wiley.

Richman, N. (1998) Looking before and after: refugees and asylum seekers in the west. In: Bracken, P.J. & Petty, C. (eds.), *Rethinking the Trauma of War*. New York: Free Association Books.

Robinson. N.S & Garber, J. (1995) Social Support and Psychopathology Across the Life Span. Perspectives on Developmental Psychopathology. In: D. Cicchetti & D.J. Cohen (eds.), *Developmental Psychopathology. Theory and Methods*, 162-213. New York: Wiley.

Rutter M. (1987) Psychological resilience and protective mechanisms. *American Journal of Orthopsychiatry 45*, 486-495.

Rutter, M. (1996) Stress research: Accomplishments and tasks ahead. In: Haggerty, R.J., Sherrod, L.R., Garmezy, N., Rutter, M. (eds.), *Stress, Risk and Resilience in Children and Adolescents*, 354-387. Cambridge: University Press.

Sveaass, N. & Reichelt, S. (2001) Refugee families in therapy: From referrals to therapeutic conversations. *Journal of Family Therapy 25*, 119-135.

Silove, D. (2000) A conceptual framework for mass trauma: implications for adaptation, intervention and debriefing. In: Raphael, B. & Wilson, J. P. (eds.), *Psychological Debriefing, Theory Practice and evidence*. Cambridge: Cambridge University Press, 337-351.

Stefanovski, G. (2004) A Tale from the Wild East. In: Snel G. (ed.), *Alter Ego. Twenty Confronting Views on the European Experience*. Amsterdam: Amsterdam University Press, 21-27.

Summerfield, D. (1997) South Africa: does a truth commission promote social reconciliation? *British Medical Journal 315,* 1393.

Summerfield, D. (1999) A critique of seven assumptions behind psychological trauma programs in war-affected areas. *Social Science & Medicine 48,* 449-1462.

De Swaan, A. (1982) *De mens is de mens een zorg.* Amsterdam: Meulenhoff.

Van der Veer, G. (1992/1998) *Counselling and Therapy with Refugees.* New York: Wiley.

Van der Veer, G. (1997) Gevluchte adolescenten. Ontwikkeling, begeleiding en hulpverlening. Utrecht: Stichting Pharos.

Van der Veer, G. (1999) Psychotherapy with traumatized refugees and asylum seekers: working through traumatic experiences or helping to cope with loneliness. *Torture 9,* 49-53.

Van Dijk, J. & Schreuder, B.J.N. (2001) De getuigenis als therapie. Beschrijving van een kortdurende therapeutische methode voor getraumatiseerde slachtoffers van politiek geweld. *Tijdschrift voor Psychotherapie 27,* 23-34.

Van Essen, J., Somers, A.G. & Bala, J. (1995). Het weven van een tapijt. Vluchtelingenkinderen en -gezinnen tussen breuk en herstel. Oorlog tekent je leven. *ICODO-Info 12,* 84-97.

Van Essen, J. (1999) Kinderen en gezinnen. In Rohlof, H., Groenenberg, M. & Bloem, C. (eds.), *Vluchtelingen in de GGZ. Handboek voor hulpverlening.* Utrecht: Stichting Pharos.

Van Essen, J. (2000) personal communication.

Walter, J. & Adam, H. (2000) Beyond victimology? Approaches and techniques for broadening up coping alternatives. In L. Van Willigen (ed.), *Heath Hazards of Organised Violence in Children II. Coping and Protective Factors,* 129-139. Utrecht: Stichting Pharos.

Walsh F. (1998). Beliefs, spirituality and transcendence: Keys to Family Resilience. In McGoldric, M, (ed.), *Re-visioning family therapy,.* 465-484. New York: The Guilford Press

Weine, S. M. (2001). Testimony with Bosnian Refugees of ethnic cleansing: Redefining merhamet after a historical nightmare. In D. Kideckel, & J. Halpern (Eds.). *War in Former Yugoslavia: Culture and Conflict.* University Park: Penn State Press.

Weingarten, K. (1998) The small and the ordinary. The daily practices of postmodern narrative therapy. *Family Process 37,* 3-15.

11. MENTAL HEALTH SERVICES IN THE UK
Lessons from transcultural psychiatry

Suman Fernando[1]

1. INTRODUCTION

The UK has seen waves of immigration over the centuries; what is relatively new for the country is that over the past forty years there has been settlement of large numbers of people whose cultural roots are from Asia, Africa and the Caribbean rather than Europe and, more importantly, of people identified as different in race to indigenous native Europeans. The terms used to describe these new groups are ethnic minorities, Black people or, more recently, Black and Asian people. As a result of strict limitations on immigration imposed in the UK and wars or ethnic conflicts outside Western Europe during the 1980s and 1990s, most recent newcomers to the country have been refugees and asylum seekers. This chapter considers some issues about the provision of mental health services for them.

For various complex reasons, mainly political in nature, British society has been conditioned to think of refugees and asylum seekers as being different in some fundamental sense to British ethnic minorities and, even when they are seen as racially non-white, to British Black people. Professionals, faced with providing mental health services appropriate to the needs of refugees and asylum seekers, have felt relatively powerless, thinking that there is insufficient information on the topic (i.e. mental health needs of refugees and asylum seekers) on which to base service delivery. Sometimes, professionals also feel inadequate in dealing with these newcomers, who are seen as having needs of a very unusual nature; they look for special training in order to provide appropriate services. In such a context, the question that needs to be addressed is whether it is an advantage or disadvantage to view refugees and asylum seekers as a separate category of people for the purpose of developing mental health services.

It is necessary to consider general ways in which refugees and asylum seekers may differ, as a group, from the majority of the indigenous British population. First, their experiences before flight in their countries of origin, and in the countries through which they may have gone during flight, may have left adverse effects on their mental health.

[1] Suman Fernando, European Centre for Migration and Social Care Studies (MASC), University of Kent, and Department of Applied Social Studies, London Metropolitan University.

Second, many would come from cultural backgrounds that are very different to that of the majority of the indigenous population and many do not speak the main language in the UK, English. Third, refugees and asylum seekers are all too often viewed with suspicion and even hostility by many people in Britain, mainly because of xenophobia – an antipathy to foreigners in general – and racism (antipathy based on skin color).

Clearly, the differences noted above would be reflected in the mental health needs of refugees and asylum seekers – needs that have to address within the services. Yet many of these differences are similar to, though not identical with, those applicable to settled ethnic minorities; and over the past twenty years an understanding has developed in some depth of mental health issues pertinent to ethnic minorities and the lessons for service provision from, what can be described as, transcultural psychiatry.

The thrust of this chapter is that, in analyzing the problems in mental health service provision, refugees should not be seen as a separate group but as basically a part of the groups we call ethnic minorities. Then, instead of professionals feeling that they cannot understand the needs of refugees until more research is carried out or – even worse – using information gathered in other places from studies that may be irrelevant or even misleading, the knowledge that already exists in the UK about the mental health field as experienced by settled ethnic minorities could come into play in arranging services that respond adequately to the challenge posed by refugees and asylum seekers.

While it is true that there may be some disadvantages in seeing refugees as part of ethnic minorities, the advantages of doing so are greater both politically (e.g. in terms of promoting their acceptance) and in organizing mental health services. It should be noted that categorization of any sort has disadvantages as well as advantages. Refugees from different parts of the world may have little in common with each other, while refugees from, say, a particular part of Africa or Asia or Eastern Europe may have quite a lot in common with settled communities from those regions. Indeed it is reasonable to assume that the outcome in terms of settlement for refugees with mental health problems would be improved if they are supported by settled communities from their own or similar background.

There have been few studies that focus on mental health of refugees after arrival in West European countries. Moreover, the results reported in these studies have to be interpreted with caution because of general methodological problems concerning Western diagnoses and test instruments applied transculturally (see Fernando, 1988, 2002; Kleinman, 1977, 1978, 1988; Weiss et al., 1995), as well as the dubious cross-cultural validity of syndromes such as PTSD (Mollica and Caspi-Yavin, 1992; Summerfield, 2000) which may be inappropriate for cross-cultural application.

Sundquist et al. (2000) studied correlations between various factors and psychological distress among refugees from Iran, Chile, Poland and Turkey between 7 and 17 years after arrival in Sweden. Their results point to risk factors for psychological distress, and to a low sense of coherence representing feelings of powerlessness and economic disadvantage in the host country, rather than adverse experiences before migration. The authors conclude that social and cultural factors in exile seem to exert a greater influence on mental health than exposure to violence before migration.

A study of Vietnamese refugees made three years after their arrival in Norway (Hauff and Vaglum, 1995) showed that the level of emotional distress did not decrease during the first years after resettlement. Many of the traumatic events experienced in Vietnam were significantly related to emotional disorder at the time of immigration to

Norway but did not show any correlation three years later. However, negative life events in Norway, lack of a close confidant, and chronic family separation were identified as predictors of psychopathology.

A study of 231 refugees referred to a psychiatric outpatient clinic in Oslo (Lavik et al., 1996) showed that 46.6% had a diagnosis of PTSD according to DSM III criteria. Torture emerged as an important predictor of emotional withdrawal/retardation but overall mental health was influenced by a variety of factors in the exile situation, such as lack of employment and educational opportunities. The authors emphasize the complexity of factors concerned with mental health of refugees and warn against generalizations.

Gorst-Unsworth and Goldenburg (1998) studied a consecutive series of 84 Iraqi refugees referred to the Medical Foundation for the Care of Victims of Torture in London between the ages of 18 and 59. They found 'considerable psychological morbidity' but no significant associations between personal trauma arising from pre-flight experiences and overall morbidity. In only 10.7% did the symptoms justify a DSM III diagnosis of PTSD although 65% had suffered systematic torture in Iraq. 45 respondents (54%) fulfilled the criteria for 'depression' as an illness; this was associated with physical torture but also with low affective support (close intimate support with an affective component unlike that provided by a professional confidant), lack of contact with a political organization, and lack of social activities after arrival in the UK. Attitudinal change – what the authors called 'existential dilemma' (Gorst-Unsworth et al., 1993) – was widely prevalent; the extent of these changes correlated not with severity of trauma but with isolation, racial attacks and dissatisfaction with housing in the host country. The overall conclusion of this British study of refugees who had faced severe persecution before arrival in England was that risk factors were multifactorial; the authors emphasized the need for integrated rehabilitation focusing on providing adequate social support and affective support from family and friends.

The general conclusions of the studies quoted above suggest that the risk to mental health has less to do with personal traumas experienced in countries of origin (although these may well be very important in the case of some individuals) and more to do with the psychosocial contexts of the lives of refugees and asylum seekers in the host country. This supports the view suggested in this chapter that information and knowledge about settled ethnic minority communities could be drawn upon in providing mental health services for refugees and asylum seekers. There is no need to assume that a new body of knowledge is required, although on-going research has a place, and certainly no need to promote a speciality in the study of refugee mental health. That is not to decry the need for professionals to be adequately trained to provide services appropriate to all sections of British society – a society that includes refugees and asylum seekers as a part of 'ethnic minority' groups. However, it must also be recognized that refugees and asylum seekers may well have specific problems and difficulties that predominate, related to their experiences immediately before migration and the specific hostility they face in the UK. From a psychological angle their sense of loss at leaving their homes of origin may well be severe and the effects of persecution by people seen by them as their kith and kin may have long term repercussions on their attitudes. Psychosocially, they may have a special need for re-integration into the community and protection from xenophobia and racism

2. MENTAL HEALTH AND ETHNIC MINORITIES IN UK

The issues around mental health highlighted in the UK over the past fifteen years are depicted in Table 1, reflecting, as it were, the tips of several icebergs of disadvantage and injustice suffered by ethnic minority ethnic groups in the UK, especially Black people.

Table 1. Racial and cultural issues: British findings.

Given High Doses of Medication

Sent to Psychiatrists by Courts

Suffer from Unmet Need

While the evidence for the problems referred to in Table 1 continues to mount, progress in addressing them has been slow and sporadic. In general the issues are those resulting from cultural diversity and racism, but the block to progress arises mainly from the latter (see Fernando, 1995). The problems within psychiatry itself (see Fernando, 1988) are compounded by wider issues (see Fernando, 2002), but there is little doubt that the problems apply to recent immigrants – refugees and asylum seekers – including those seen as white.

2.1. Racism in Practice

Britain has always been a culturally diverse society and what has happened over the past few years is that attitudes towards cultural diversity have become complicated by attitudes about race – by racism. And for refugees and asylum seekers, political and legal issues have further complicated matters. The very definition of refugee or asylum seeker is a legal and political one and not one of health status. The negative stereotypes and racist attitudes that are now recognized as causing some of the problems that Black and Asian people in Britain have in deriving appropriate help from mental health services are, if anything, aggravated for refugees and asylum seekers.

It has been said that racism is no longer seen in its most blatant overt form in the UK but that subtle racism through unwitting behavior and institutionalized ways of doing things is the main problem. However, some of the statements made recently about refugees and asylum seekers by important politicians and some sections of the media indicate that overt racism is not dead. But returning to the concept of subtle racism, much of this appears to be institutionalized in training and education. On the whole, the training of professionals working in the mental health field and with refugees in general instills a (quite unrealistic and racist) confidence in the superiority over all others of the body of knowledge and ways of working within Western disciplines that inform our systems of care – psychiatry and psychology certainly, but also counseling and psychotherapy.

In practice, mental health assessments usually fail to allow for ideologies about life, approaches to life's problems, beliefs and feelings that come from non-Western cultures. The causes of justified anger arising from racism in society are often not recognized because the black experience – especially the experience of racism – in society is not given credence, even if the existence of personal discrimination is recognized in a theoretical sort of way. The alienation felt by most black people – and by refugees – is usually seen as *their* problem, and this often leads to treatment aimed at getting people to recognize reality rather than treating it as a problem for society as a whole. And when the experiences and feelings of black people are recognized as significant, a disease or criminal model is used to conceptualize them, because society and possibly our own needs promote this. In such a context, stereotypical assumptions influence assessments that professionals make. The report of an inquiry into the deaths of three black men who died in Broadmoor Hospital (Special Hospitals Service Authority (SHSA), 1993) called for research into the problem created by the stereotype 'big, black and dangerous'.

The racial bias of the psychiatric process is so much a part of its central core that it is difficult to know how to separate it from Western psychiatry, to say nothing of eliminating it. And such bias applies to other fields in mental health apart from psychiatry – for example, psychotherapy and counseling. Psychiatric diagnoses carry their own special images, which may connect up with other images derived from common sense. 'Schizophrenia' is diagnosed 10 to 20 times more frequently among Black people compared to Whites, more so in those born in Britain than among immigrants (see e.g. Harrison et al., 1988). And this when, even from a purely medical angle, the validity – the usefulness – of diagnoses such as schizophrenia have not been shown in a transcultural context.

Diagnoses are too often influenced by – indeed dependent on – images and models carried in people's minds, perpetuated by theory and research, and reflected in stereotypes and attitudes (Fernando, 1988). Thus, alienness seems to be linked to schizophrenia, as a diagnosis and to biological and/or cultural inferiority, as a judgment that is often implicit, rather than explicit. Race comes into both these concepts – alienness and inferiority. In a setting of psychiatric practice where the difference between treatment and control is seldom very clear, and where mental health professionals may be faced with people who do not fit into the traditional norms delineated in textbooks or present as frightening or dangerous, distorted assessments are made and inappropriate diagnoses given in order to control.

The matter of 'dangerousness' has become a topical issue ion recent years, with repeated attempts by the UK government to remodel mental health legislation to address 'the safety of the public'. Psychiatrists and psychologists have little to go on, yet they make assessments of dangerousness using common-sense images of dangerous people as a guide – and within such common sense are prejudices and assumptions reflecting those in society at large. Indeed, dangerousness and schizophrenia appear to be conflated in the minds of both lay people and many psychiatrists. Moreover, racist images are implicated in both.

3. MENTAL HEALTH AND CULTURAL DIVERSITY

Although Britain today is multi-ethnic, the mental health services are largely under the influence of Western psychiatry and psychology, which in turn are informed by narrow traditions derived mainly from traditional European roots. In other words, mental health services are monocultural, meaning that the professionals who staff them come from a culture – a culture of training – which is primarily based on Western ways of analyzing human problems, determining what is health and illness, etc. The services thus reflect concepts about health and illness drawn from cultural models that are inappropriate for a multicultural society. Furthermore, for historical reasons, the services reflect ways of thinking and working, attitudes and assumptions, fears and prejudices, all of which go to form what is generally referred to as 'institutional racism'. So in short, British society is multicultural and multiracial while the mental health services are ethnocentric or monocultural and, generally speaking, racist.

Concerning cultural differences we can say, speaking very generally, that in Eastern traditions health is regarded as a harmonious balance between various forces in the person and the social context. For example, the Chinese way of thinking sees all illness as an imbalance of *yin* and *yang*; two complementary poles of life energy, to be corrected by attempts to re-establish balance (Aakster, 1986). The Indian tradition emphasizes the harmony between the person and his/her group as indicative of health (Kakar, 1982); and the concept of health in African culture is more social than biological (Lambo, 1969). In all these non-Western cultures, human life is conceptualized as an indivisible whole that includes not just 'mind' and 'body' as one, but also the spiritual dimension of human life. Further, understanding of the human condition does not in non-Western cultures naturally divide up into the fields of study of psychology, religion and philosophy as defined in the West. Indeed studying the minds of human beings separately from their bodies and spirits, as psychology does, and interpreting human problems concerning thinking, beliefs, emotions and feelings, etc. in illness terms, as psychiatry does, may seem very odd – and very confusing – to someone with a holistic worldview. Eastern and Western ideals of mental health are contrasted for purposes of this argument in Table 2. (Fernando, 1995).

In considering treatment for problems interpreted in Western terms as mental, the Western tradition of psychology and psychiatry sees therapy as a process apart from both the therapist and the client receiving the therapy. Table 3. (Fernando, 1995) contrasts Eastern and Western approaches to therapy. In a cultural setting where problems conceptualized as mental in the West are seen as spiritual experiences or ethical dilemmas, the process of dealing with them – or coping with the distress caused by them – is not therapy in a Western sense. The usual term used may be akin to liberation from distress; techniques are less separable from the person or persons involved. Western approaches can be seen as focused on control of, for example, symptoms, or understanding by analysis in, for example, psychotherapy. In cultures that emphasize harmony, balance and integration within the individual, acceptance of problems or symptoms is more important than control, and understanding by contemplation supersedes the need to analyze feelings.

The contents of Table 2 and Table 3 should not be seen in black and white terms – in any sense of the words. As Sudhir Kakar (1982) says, the terms East and West indicate states of mind rather than geographical regions. Contrasting East with West should not be

Table 2. Ideals of mental health.

EASTERN	WESTERN
Integration and Harmony	**Self-sufficiency**
* **Between Person and Environment** * **Between Families** * **Within Societies** * **In relation to spiritual values**	
Social Integration	**Personal Autonomy**
Balanced Functioning	**Efficiency**
Protection and Caring	**Self Esteem**

Table 3. Approaches to therapy.

EASTERN	WESTERN
Acceptance	**Control**
Harmony	**Personal Autonomy**
Understanding by Awareness	**Understanding by analysis**
Contemplation	**Problem Solving**
Body-Mind-Spirit Unity	**Body-Mind separate**

seen as an attempt to reduce complex varieties of culturally determined world views to simple categories, but merely as a simplification of these for the purposes of this discussion. The differences that are identified represent frames of reference rather than absolute entities. Moreover, there is a large overlap between cultural groups and there is constant interchange of ideas and influences (although power, prestige and economic advantage rather than validity affect these). The themes represent overall ideologies that underpin people's lives, rather than intellectual views.

A point that needs to be made at this stage is that education and training, for example in psychotherapy, derived from Western sources are underpinned by Western ways of thinking and many professionals trained in such systems make assumptions based on their 'obvious' superiority, scientific worth etc., reflecting cultural arrogance, reflecting racism.

4. CONCLUSIONS

It is argued in this chapter that refugees and asylum seekers should be seen as ethnic minorities for the purpose of planning mental health services, although it is acknowledged that there are specific issues that apply to them – in particular, those concerning their pre-flight experiences. There is sufficient information on the issues around racism and cultural diversity that impinge upon the provision of mental health services in the UK to enable services to be planned that are appropriate for a multicultural and multi-ethnic society – for a society that addresses the needs of ethnic minorities, whether they are living in settled communities or are recent arrivals. However it should be noted that refugees from different countries might have very little in common with each other in terms of pre-flight experiences. So lumping together all refugees and looking for solutions to refugee problems may be too limited an approach.

The need for ethnic monitoring of mental health services is well recognized. In view of the fact that most recent arrivals are refugees and asylum seekers, ethnic monitoring must be supplemented by routine monitoring of refugee/asylum seeker status indicating origin. Services need to be supported by an easily accessible interpreter service covering all the languages that may be encountered. Indeed, refugees themselves may well be able to participate in such a service with some training in the use of English. Professionals may well need on-going support – and refugee organizations in the area served may well be able to provide this. The limitations of Western diagnostic models, methods of assessment and Western concepts of therapy need to be addressed in service provision and it should be appreciated that racism affects the practice of psychiatry, psychotherapy etc. The problems for ethnic minorities that have arisen from the uncritical use of schizophrenia as a diagnosis are likely to apply to refugees too. There is considerable evidence (see Summerfield, 2000) that the use of PTSD as a diagnosis to conceptualize mental health problems of refugees and asylum seekers may play a similar role. Indeed the use of this diagnosis, except in a few carefully selected instances, in the case of refugees and asylum seekers arriving in Western Europe may result in detracting from a proper understanding of their mental health needs, which are usually varied and multifactorial.

The most important point to emerge from the experience of ethnic minorities is that the voices of the communities themselves – the people who are potential users of the service – must be properly heard. Refugees and asylum seekers should not be treated as passive recipients of services, but as active participants who have a wealth of knowledge about their needs and the sort of assistance they require in order to re-build their lives in a new country. Services need to be sufficiently flexible so that any help they receive should be able to build upon their own way of coping consistent with their cultural backgrounds. It is important to bear in mind that refugees are generally highly resourceful people who have encountered and overcome many problems.

REFERENCES

Aakster, C. W. (1986) Concepts in alternative medicine. *Social Science and Medicine 22*, 265-273.

Eisenbruch, M. (1991) From Post-Traumatic Stress Disorder to Cultural Bereavement: Diagnosis of Southeast Asian Refugees. *Social Science and Medicine 33*, 673-680.

Fernando, S. (1988) *Race and Culture in Psychiatry.* London: Croom Helm. Paperback edition, London: Routledge, 1989.

Fernando, S. (1995a) Social realities and mental health. In: S. Fernando (ed.), *Mental Health in a Multi-ethnic Society. A Multidisciplinary Handbook.* London: Routledge, 11-35.

Fernando, S. (1995b) Professional interventions; therapy and care. In: S. Fernando (ed.), *Mental Health in a Multi-ethnic Society. A Multidisciplinary Handbook.* London: Routledge, 36-49.

Fernando, S. (2002) *Mental Health, Race and Culture,* Second Edition. London: Palgrave.

Gorst-Unsworth, C., Van Velsen, C. & Turner, S. W. (1993) Prospective pilot study of survivors of torture and organised violence. Examining the existential dilemma. *Journal of Nervous and Mental Disease 181*, 263-264.

Gorst-Unsworth, C. and Goldenberg, E. (1998) Psychological sequelae of torture and organised violence suffered by refugees from Iraq. Trauma related factors compared with social factors in exile. *British Journal of Psychiatry 172*, 90-94.

Harrison, G., Owens, D., Holton, A., Neilson, D. and Boot, D. (1988) A prospective study of severe mental disorder in Afro-Caribbean patients. *Psychological Medicine 18*, 643-57.

Hauff, E. and Vaglum, P. (1995, Organised violence and the stress of exile. Predictors of mental health in a community cohort of Vietnamese refugees three years after resettlement. *British Journal of Psychiatry 166*, 360-367.

Kakar, S. (1982) *Shamans, Mystics and Doctors.* London: Unwin.

Kleinman, A. (1977) Depression, somatization and the 'new cross-cultural psychiatry'. *Social Science and Medicine 11*, 3-10.

Kleinman, A. (1978) Concepts and a model for the comparison of medical systems as cultural systems. *Social Science and Medicine 12*, 85-93.

Kleinman, A. (1988) *Rethinking Psychiatry. From Cultural Category to Personal Experience.* New York: The Free Press.

Lambo, A. (1969) Traditional African cultures and Western medicine. In F. N. L. Poynter (ed.), *Medicine and Culture.* London: Welcome Institute for History of Medicine.

Lavik, N. J., Hauff, E., Skrondal, A. and Solberg, O. (1996) Mental Disorder among refugees and the impact of persecution and exile: some findings from an out-patient population. *British Journal of Psychiatry 169*, 726-732.

Mollica, R. F. and Caspi-Yavin, Y. (1992) Overview: The assessment and diagnosis of torture events and symptoms. In M. Basoglu (ed.), *Torture and its consequences: current treatment approaches.* Cambridge: Cambridge University Press, 253-274.

Pourgourides, C. K., Sashidharan, S. P. and Bracken, P. J. (1996) *A Second Exile. The Mental Health Implications of Detention of Asylum Seekers in the United Kingdom.* Birmingham: The University of Birmingham and The Barrow Cadbury Trust.

Special Hospitals Service Authority (SHSA) (1993) *Report of the Committee of Inquiry into the Death in Broadmoor Hospital of Orville Blackwood and a Review of the Deaths of Two Other Afro-Caribbean Patients: 'Big, Black and Dangerous?',* Chairman Professor H. Prins. London: SHSA.

Summerfield, D. (2000) War and Mental Health *British Medical Journal 321*, 232-235.

Sundquist, J., Bayard-Burfield, L., Johansson, L. M. and Johansson, S. (2000) Impact of ethnicity, violence and acculturation on displaced migrants. Psychological distress and psychosomatic complaints among refugees in Sweden. *Journal of Nervous and Mental Disease 188*, 357-365.

Weiss, M. G., Raguram, R. and Channabasavanna (1995) Cultural dimensions of psychiatric diagnosis. Comparison of DSM-III-R and illness explanatory models in South India. *British Journal of Psychiatry* *166*, 353-359.

Young, A. (1995) *The Harmony of Illusions. Inventing Post-Traumatic Stress Disorder.* Princeton, NY: Princeton University Press.

12. MENTAL HEALTH AND SOCIAL CARE FOR ASYLUM SEEKERS AND REFUGEES
A comparative study

David Ingleby and Charles Watters[1]

1. INTRODUCTION

This chapter describes the results of a study (Watters et al., 2003) which was carried out for the European Commission (European Refugee Fund) during 2002 and 2003. The aim of the project was to promote the international exchange of good practice, experience and expertise concerning interventions aimed at the psychosocial well-being of asylum seekers and refugees. The project contained two elements. One, the 'identification study', was concerned with making an inventory of practices in selected countries. Alongside this, the 'implementation study' set out to transfer promising interventions from one country to another.

The following considerations motivated this project. In recent years, countries in Europe have been faced with the challenge of providing adequate health and social care for growing numbers of asylum-seekers and refugees. Despite the many problems for which the latter are 'at risk', their access to services may be impeded by a variety of factors. In addition, the help they receive may be less than optimal. Professionals often lack the training and experience necessary to recognize and deal with the specific needs of this group, while cultural and language differences may exacerbate problems of service delivery.

In response to such problems, agencies all over the world have devoted considerable effort to developing expertise and 'good practices' in this area. To date, however, this has mostly been done within the borders of each country: there has been little systematic international exchange of experience. This project examined the problems of identifying good practices and facilitating their transfer between countries. We believe that the best way forward in this field, as in most others, is through an international exchange of ideas. Innovations pioneered in one country may never have been considered in another; effort

[1] David Ingleby, Faculty of Social Sciences, Utrecht University, The Netherlands.
Charles Watters, European Centre for Migration and Social Care Studies (MASC), University of Kent, UK.

may be wasted in one country on developing interventions which elsewhere have been shown to be flawed.

Transferring good practices from one country to another involves the following steps. Firstly, successful interventions must be identified. Secondly, the differences between the context within which such 'good practices' were developed, and the one in which they will be applied, must be examined. Thirdly, in the light of this, the practices have to be adapted to the new context. Fourthly, information about the practices has to be disseminated; and fifthly, they must be implemented. Since it would have taken too long to carry out all these steps sequentially, we divided the process into two sub-projects. The 'identification study' dealt with the first two steps, while the 'implementation study' covered the last three.

1.1. Background of the study

Between 1983 and 1992 there was a tenfold increase in asylum applications in Western Europe (from 70,000 to 700,000). The surge in the early 1990's was due to the Balkans wars; over the last ten years refugees also came from Romania, Turkey, Iraq, Afghanistan, Sri Lanka, Iran, Somalia, the Congo and many other countries. After reaching a peak in 1992 the number of asylum seekers started to decline, reaching 245,000 in 1996. This decline was partly due to a lull in the Balkans conflict, but also to the adoption of increasingly stringent procedures for the admission of asylum seekers and the granting of refugee status. Since the mid-nineties, countries of the industrialized world have vied with each other in developing the most restrictive asylum policy.

The provision of effective health and social care for asylum seekers and refugees is partly motivated by principles of human rights, and partly by pragmatic considerations. The right to care is laid down in the 1951 Geneva Convention on Refugees; more recently, the European Commission adopted on 27th January 2003 a directive laying down minimum standards on the reception of asylum applicants in Member States, including standards of health care. But apart from the question of human rights, governments also have an interest in ensuring that this group is not neglected. Ignoring the problems people have usually leads to more serious problems at a later stage. For example, a refugee handicapped by psychosocial problems is likely to have difficulty getting a job and integrating into the host society, thereby becoming even more dependent on the state.

There are two arenas in which care may be provided: locally, within the conflict region (for example in temporary refugee camps), and in host countries within the developed world. In conflict regions, help is usually provided by internationally funded NGO's. The present study is primarily concerned with the provision of services in host countries. Here, the established services have to deal with problems and client populations with which they are unfamiliar. Our research shows that giving refugees the formal right to care is one thing: ensuring that the care is accessible and effective is quite another.

2. DESIGN OF PROJECT AND THEORETICAL APPROACH

2.1. Aims of the two sub-projects

2.1.1. The identification study

This part of the project was concerned with identifying good practices and characterizing the context in which they have been developed. We chose to study in detail two Northern European countries (the United Kingdom and The Netherlands) and two Southern European ones (Spain and Portugal). During 2002, the number of asylum applications in these countries was as follows: United Kingdom 110,700; Netherlands 18,567; Spain 5,179; and Portugal 245 (UNHCR, 2003). The low figures for Spain and (especially) Portugal may be deceptive: they conceal the fact that the category of 'illegal aliens' probably harbors many fleeing from danger or persecution who are unwilling or unable to enter the asylum procedure, or who have been rejected by it.

The suitability of an intervention for transfer depends not only on its quality, but also on its appropriateness in the new context. There are important differences between countries concerning the context in which services have been developed. These include social and political attitudes to issues of asylum and immigration, structures and traditions of care, and the size and composition of the refugee population. Often interventions will need to be drastically modified to suit the conditions obtaining in another country, while some may be simply non-transferable.

Besides the four 'country reports' mentioned above, a fifth survey dealt with interventions developed in Australia, Canada and Guatemala. Because of the limitations of this part of the study, its results are not described in this chapter. Interested readers are referred to the full version of the research report.

2.1.2. The implementation study

This part of the project was 'action research', aimed at gathering concrete experience of the obstacles which may be encountered when attempting to transfer interventions between countries. We chose interventions which could be regarded as relatively successful in their country of origin. To increase the chances of success, we also chose a pair of countries offering similar contexts: the UK and the Netherlands. The many resemblances between the mental health care services and professional philosophies in these two countries have been documented in Gijswijt-Hofstra and Porter (1996). New legislation introduced in Britain in 2000 meant that both countries had a policy of dispersing of asylum-seekers nationwide. They also relied mainly on existing services to provide care.

In both countries, we selected an intervention which was highly regarded by experts in the field and had been positively evaluated, but had received little consideration in the other country. We attempted to initiate the transfer of these practices and observed the difficulties which can arise in practice when attempting to transfer practices which are highly promising in theory.

- The British intervention which was considered for transfer to the Netherlands was the 'Breathing Space' project (see Watters, 2001). This is a collaboration between the Refugee Council and the Medical Foundation, financed by the Camelot Foundation, which aims to address the different needs of refugees and asylum seekers in a coordinated way.

- The Dutch intervention consisted of a package of programs for school-age children of refugees and asylum seekers, developed by the Pharos Foundation with the aim of facilitating integration and adjustment and helping to prevent psychosocial problems (see Ingleby and Watters, 2002).

2.2. Clarification of key concepts

2.2.1. The notion of 'good practice'

In the case of mental health and social care for refugees, defining 'good practice' is not simply a matter of quantifying the effectiveness of a particular intervention in solving problems. Evaluation in this setting is much more complex and many-dimensional than, say, assessing different techniques for replacing hip joints. In the care for refugees, questions of accessibility, good communication and trust in the help offered are crucially important factors alongside the effectiveness of a given procedure in purely clinical terms.

As Watters (2001) has described, there are conflicting and competing paradigms or schools of thought regarding the way in which refugees' problems should be viewed and dealt with. Because we were dealing with a field which is complex and in certain respects contentious, we decided to adopt broad definitions of problems and treatments and not to impose a fictive consensus on the field when it comes to defining the 'state of the art'. One option would have been to take the problem constructions and working methods of health service providers as a given, and simply to ask the question: "what services are available for refugees suffering from (for example) PTSD, and how effective are they?" However, to do so would have been to align our research too closely with the frame of reference of the service providers themselves, which may be quite different from that of the users. We have therefore chosen broad definitions of problems, services, practices and criteria for 'good practice'. Our results provide, at most, a starting-point for more intensive future studies concerned with the quality of service provision for this group.

2.2.2. Which problems?

Western professionals in the fields of mental health and social care tend to see psychosocial problems as distinct from material, social or political problems on the one hand, and somatic ones on the other. Within these boundaries, the category comprises problems which range from psychiatric disorders to 'normal reactions to abnormal situations'. Many users, on the other hand, may not share these categories or even be aware of their existence. As Suman Fernando pointed out in Chapter 11, they may not be in the habit of separating 'internal' problems from 'external' ones, or experiencing their mind and body as separate. Instead, they may view psychological, material, social, political and somatic problems as inseparable. As a result, they may not locate problems 'in' the individual, or regard individual treatment as an appropriate response to them. To use Arthur Kleinman's terminology (1981), their 'explanatory models' may not match those of the professionals. Since the users' perspective is important to us, so are these discrepancies.

However, since this research was concerned with improvements to the care system, it could not afford to ignore professional notions. We therefore opted for a pragmatic approach, in which attention was paid to the perspectives of both professionals and users.

2.2.3. Which services?

We also did not want to limit the research to mental health care organizations and social work departments. Sometimes, interventions aimed at psychological well-being are carried out by professionals working outside the mental health system (e.g. school counselors). Interventions may also be carried out by non-professionals.

Prevention is also an aspect of care, and many sorts of intervention not regarded as 'mental health and social care' can have an impact on psychosocial problems. For example, recreational activities or language courses can improve refugees' abilities to cope. This creates a difficult boundary problem: the range of activities which can influence a refugee's state of psychological well-being is theoretically enormous. Does the removal of a repressive regime by military means be categorized as 'preventive mental health work'? Most would say no - but lobbying against stressful asylum procedures, unjustified detention and humiliating treatment can indeed be viewed as part of the professional responsibility of those concerned with refugee mental health (see Chapter 1). Nevertheless, it would have made the scope of this research impossibly broad to examine everything which could be regarded as a preventive activity. We have therefore confined this concept to *activities which define their own goals in such terms.*

2.2.4. Which practices?

What counts as a 'practice'? The most obvious level concerns treatment ('primary process'). However, many working in this field do not describe their own activities as 'treatment'. Moreover, the accessibility of a service, its closeness to users' culture and life world and the way it is organized, are also highly relevant to is effectiveness. In this study we decided to distinguish the following four major aspects of service provision:

- Organizational changes: these do not concern so much the type of help that is given, as the way service provision is organized. Relevant issues are: where are services located? How are they financed? How (if at all) are their activities coordinated? What is done to improve the standards of service on a national level? Are there agencies which consolidate and disseminate existing knowledge and develop new knowledge?
- Training and education: improving the expertise of health and social care workers is a vital foundation for 'good practice'.
- Treatment: this may be given within the context of regular care, or as part of a special facility.
- Preventive activities. These activities are especially important within the public health or mental hygiene perspectives described in Chapter 1.

2.2.5. Criteria for good practice

Assessing service provision in this area is, as we have seen, a complex matter. It is also subject to many practical and methodological pitfalls. For example, many interventions involve small numbers and a client population which is extremely difficult to trace and follow up. Ethical, organizational or financial considerations often make it virtually impossible to set up controlled clinical trials with an experimental design. Problems of sampling bias and inadequate cross-cultural validity of the instruments to be used are also endemic.

Apart from controlled clinical trials, however, there are other types of evaluation which may fare better. *Process evaluation* gathers information about whether an intervention does what it sets out to do and whether it reaches, and holds, the target group. The *satisfaction* of both caregivers and users can be assessed. However, these data are harder to interpret, for at least two reasons. One is that answers may reflect strategic considerations (e.g. not wanting to 'let the side down' or to appear difficult; wanting to ensure that an activity is continued). The other is that it is quite possible for a genuine feeling of satisfaction to accompany a treatment which entirely fails to improve the condition it set out to improve - and vice versa.

Another form of evaluation, *plan evaluation,* can be carried out even before an intervention has been put into practice. To what extent does the intervention take account of well-known pitfalls and shortcomings of the type of activity in question? Does it appear to be informed by the current 'state of the art'? A problem with plan evaluation, however, is that different schools of thought may prioritize goals which are actually in conflict with each other. A recent example is the reorganization of youth services in the Netherlands. To improve the 'professionalism' of these services, systematic procedures were introduced based on the model of clinical practice. This entailed closing low-threshold, informal 'walk-in' centers where young people could drop in and air their problems informally and discretely, as well as many 'outreaching' programs. The result was a service with stricter standards and procedures, but one which was effectively inaccessible to many of its intended users.

In this study, most of our effort went into simply making an inventory of existing practices. Where possible, we included data on process evaluation, satisfaction and effectiveness evaluation, but this was seldom available. In selecting promising innovations, we therefore paid attention to questions such as these:

- How *accessible* is the intervention?

- How are the needs or wishes of users reflected in the intervention?

- Have users influenced, directly or indirectly, the form of the activity?

- How much attention is paid to possible effects of cultural differences?

- Is the intervention *original?*

- Are attempts made to *evaluate* the success of the intervention?

3. METHODS

3.1. Identification study

For each of the countries studied, an overview was made of the size and nature of the refugee and asylum-seeker population in each land, their particular needs, the services available for dealing with them, the problems arising in service delivery and the methods adopted for dealing with these problems. In order to facilitate comparisons, a more or less standardized 'template' was used to gather information. This template was adapted in the course of the investigation to accommodate new insights.

For most of these questions, secondary sources could be used, although occasionally the project carried out its own research (e.g. on service provisions in the UK and on problems experienced by migrants and service providers in Portugal). Much information was provided by the collaborating agencies in each land. In addition, unpublished documents were located and expert opinions obtained.

The information gathered was placed in the context of the distinctive political, demographic and cultural features of each country. The Canterbury research team covered the UK and Spain, while the Utrecht team carried out the same task for The Netherlands and Portugal. Both teams gathered information on non-EU countries. Findings were presented for critical review to experts in each country and amended in accordance with their comments.

At the end of the project, a conference was held in Brussels at which participants from the main countries studied exchanged views on the results and helped to formulate the conclusions of the report.

3.2. Implementation study

Firstly, the experience gathered on the two selected practices was summarized. Both had been subject to evaluations in which strong and weak points had been identified. Next, differences in the context of service provision within different countries were analyzed which might make modification necessary. Proposals were made for modifying the practices to make them suitable for transfer.

After this, a manual summarizing the results of these steps was produced. Drafts of this manual were submitted for critical assessment and feedback to selected experts familiar with the interventions. After revision, the manuals were sent to the research team in the other country as a basis for taking the project further.

This team then organized expert meetings with key stakeholders to discuss the best strategy for implementing it the projects On the basis of these meetings, a strategy for implementation was outlined and the researchers proceeded as far as possible with piloting and evaluating the intervention in question.

Finally, the success of the transfer was evaluated and recommendations were made about continuation, modification or termination of the innovation.

4. RESULTS

4.1. Identification Study

The four main 'country reports' were built up as described below. The numbering of the paragraphs in the summaries of these reports corresponds to the chapters listed here. The reports on Australia, Canada and Guatemala were less detailed and highlighted particularly innovative or successful interventions.

Table 1. Structure of country reports.

Chapter 1. The context of interventions
Demographic and political aspects of immigration. Main groups of immigrants; public attitudes; immigration and asylum policy; the role of the media; procedures for admission, reception and accommodation of asylum seekers. Rights and restrictions applying to this group.
Needs and problems of asylum seekers and refugees (combining official and professional views with the perspective of the groups themselves, on the basis of published research, interviews with group members, and other informants).

Chapter 2. Mental health and social care provisions
Short sketch of the care system, with special attention to mental health services. Historical background, financing and organizational structure. Social and community care, forms of health and social care offered outside the regular framework by NGO's (including religious bodies) and self-help organizations.
Multicultural care provisions. The 'state of the art' in multicultural service provisions, with special attention to mental health. What problems have arisen in service provision for migrants, and what solutions have been offered so far?
Services for asylum seekers and refugees. To what sorts of care are asylum seekers and refugees entitled? How accessible are these care provisions? What problems have arisen?

Chapter 3. Practices developed for asylum seekers and refugees
Inventory of practices. What solutions have been developed so far? What are the philosophies underlying these innovations? Practices were classified according to the categories described above (Organizational changes, training and education, treatment, preventive activities).

Chapter 4. Good practices
Summary of strong and weak points of service provision. Case studies (detailed description of individual projects or approaches which are felt to be particularly innovative and promising).

4.1.1. United Kingdom

(1) Historically, much of the immigration to the United Kingdom has been connected with the country's imperial past. Substantial immigration took place in the second half of the 20th century, and much of this concerned inhabitants of the former colonies (the major groups being West Indians, Pakistanis and Indians). The UK also recruited cheap labor from the rest of Europe during the economic expansion of the 1950's and 1960's. At the present time, Britain's major cities house large communities of immigrants, and around 8,4% of the total population is foreign born or born in the UK to foreign-born parents.

Since 1965, a series of Race Relations Acts have been passed to control racism and discrimination. Although immigration controls are tight, government policy is overtly multicultural and stresses the contribution made by immigrants to the nation. Nevertheless, racial tensions are a constant source of concern in British politics.

Up to the end of the 1980's, asylum applications numbered only two or three thousand annually. In 1991 this total had increased to nearly fifty thousand, mainly because of the Balkans conflict; 2001 saw a total of 71,700 applications. Thus, Britain has become one of the major European countries receiving asylum seekers. In 2001, 74% of these applications were refused. Major legislative changes governing asylum policy were passed in 1993, 1996, 1999 and 2002, reflecting the difficulties the UK had in adapting to this relatively large influx. As we also noted in the Netherlands and Spain, the end of the 1990's ushered in a period of increasingly negative presentation of asylum seekers (and immigrants in general) in the media.

After the reception phase, asylum seekers are dispersed to areas all over the UK. This policy was introduced in 2000 to counter the large concentration of asylum seekers in the South East and London. Accommodation arrangements are varied; there are few large-scale centers, but the used of detention in prisons or prison-like facilities has become a controversial feature of British policy.

Many of the needs and problems of asylum seekers in Britain are connected with government policy and public attitudes. The dispersal policy undermines informal support networks and hampers integration. Living conditions are often experienced as stressful. Discrimination and public hostility can also exacerbate these stresses. Quite apart from this, of course, many asylum seekers also have psychological problems as a result of their pre-flight experiences, as well as the worries and uncertainties associated with living in exile.

(2) Health care in the UK is provided by the National Health Service and is free at the point of supply. The general practitioner (GP) functions as the main 'gatekeeper' to the health care system. Asylum seekers are entitled to make use of the NHS, though the difference between *rights* and *access* is highlighted by the difficulty asylum seekers can experience in getting on to a GP's list.

Mental health care services are provided by local Community Mental Health Teams (CMHT's), which aim to offer integrated, 'joined-up' health care in which social and practical problems are considered in relation to mental and physical ones.

There is little systematic, structural attention to the problems of multicultural mental health care delivery in the UK, yet there is much expertise to be found and there are many local initiatives. In the remote areas to which asylum seekers are often dispersed, however, service providers may be totally unused to dealing with clients with a different cultural background.

(3) To identify promising practices, the researchers undertook a survey of service providers, identifying 59 which were active in developing care for asylum seekers and refugees. 80% of these were in London. 26 services replied to a postal questionnaire and of these, 14 showed elements of good practice, in terms of accessibility, user involvement, multi-agency linkages, continuity of services and care, cultural sensitivity, advocacy, evaluation and research. The research identified both structural innovations and innovations in the field of therapy. Training and education for professionals working with refugees and/or migrants is not widely available, but some programs exist. Preventive activities are organized by some local authorities and by NGO's such as the Refugee Council, which provide various support and advisory services.

(4) The report singled out three especially promising innovations as examples of good practices. The first was a specialized GP service for newly arrived and resident asylum seekers and refugees, located close to a major port of arrival. In London, the Bayswater Family Center provided comprehensive family support to homeless and refugee families. Both these services had a range of multi-agency linkages. Finally, a preventive project in the North of England was described, which used gardening as a means of recreation and social contact. This project had been highly rated by users.

In this context we should also mention the 'bi-cultural team' of the 'Breathing Space' project, a London-based intake and referral program described below in the results of the Implementation Study.

4.1.2. The Netherlands

(1) The context of interventions in the Netherlands is in many respects similar to that in the UK. In the second half of the 20th century, the main immigrant groups consisted of people born in the former Dutch colonies and labor migrants, the largest groups being from Turkey and Morocco. Through family reunification and reproduction, the latter have come to number more than 600.000 (about 4% of the total population). Since the 1970's, Dutch policy on admitting non-Western labor migrants has been restrictive.

The number of asylum applications to the Netherlands increased by a factor of twenty (from 2,603 to 52,570) between 1984 and 1994, and throughout the 1990's, the Netherlands remained (in proportion to its own population) one of the major European asylum countries, along with the UK and Germany. However, recent years saw the introduction of stricter admission policies: in 2002 the figure had dropped back to 18,667.

Historically speaking, Dutch attitudes to ethnic diversity were for a long time notably liberal. This tradition goes back to the 16th and 17th century: it was reinforced by the German occupation of 1940-1945, which strengthened hostility to racism and persecution. The Dutch government formally adopted a policy of 'multiculturalism' at the beginning of the 1980's.

In recent years, however – as in other European countries – a different wind has been blowing. Hostility has increased towards people of Turkish and (especially) Moroccan origin, who are accused of 'backwardness' and inadequate integration. The populist politician Pim Fortuyn campaigned for the 2002 elections on a platform with included a complete ban on immigration. Since his assassination in that year, his ideas have formed the core of a xenophobic revival, leading to measures against immigrants and asylum seekers which have earned the Netherlands complaints by human rights organizations.

Asylum procedures were modified continually during the last 15 years, but the underlying principle has remained unchanged that most asylum seekers are accommodated in special centers that are spread over the whole country. Processing of applications often takes several years, during which period rights to work and education are very limited. All these circumstances are reported by asylum seekers to give rise to considerable stress.

(2) The inhabitants of The Netherlands enjoy a high standard of health and social care is also of a high standard. Health care is based on a mixed system, run partly by the state and partly by private organizations. Alongside compulsory state medical insurance, one-third of the population is insured with private companies. As in Britain, the government hopes that the operation of market forces will lead to increased efficiency and reduction of costs. Care provisions in the Netherlands are characterized by a high degree of professionalization, though some work is still carried out by voluntary organizations (in particular, the advisory services for refugees provided by Vluchtelingenwerk)

The general practitioner plays a central role in Dutch health care, since he or she provides access to other parts of the health care system and is the point of referral. The mental health care system was strongly influenced by American models of 'community care'.

For some 25 years, a small but active group of professionals has called attention to the problems of service provision for migrants and ethnic minorities. During this period many initiatives have been sent up, mostly on a short-term, project basis. Awareness of the issues is fairly widespread, especially in the big cities (where more than half of the young adult population is often of foreign extraction). However, it was not until 2000 that the government acknowledged the need for structural measures. As a result of the drastic shift to the right in Dutch politics, active support for 'interculturalization' seems now to have been withdrawn.

Health care for refugees was originally provided mainly within the accommodation centers themselves, but there has been an increasing tendency to incorporate it within the regular system. From 2000, mental health care for asylum seekers was entirely delegated to the regular service providers. Since 1993 the "Pharos Foundation for Refugees and Health", funded by the government, has been responsible for furthering expertise in the care for this group. Refugees and asylum seekers enjoy virtually the same rights to health care as other inhabitants of the Netherlands; however, problems of access and effectiveness remain.

(2) A large number of innovations (68) were identified in our search for 'good practices'. This reflects the fact that refugees have received systematic attention from professionals in the Netherlands, which – until recently – was one of the major destinations for asylum seekers. Expertise centers (Pharos and Mikado) have been set up for the care of refugees and migrants. Other organizational innovations have concerned unaccompanied minors and victims of sexual violence. Alongside this, networks or consultation schemes have been set up to improve and coordinate refugee health care.

There are also a fair number of training and education programs, many of them organized by Pharos. Concerning treatment, seven specialized clinics, centers or programs for refugees were identified: twelve other initiatives concerned specialized forms of treatment. An particularly large number of practices (27) concerned prevention, most being carried out by agencies or groups outside the regular health care system.

Our report concluded that in the Netherlands, "the challenge of providing care to asylum seekers and refugees has stimulated a great deal of innovative activity at all levels - from government departments and service providers to voluntary organizations". Among the organizational innovations, we singled out *expertise centers* and *attempts to improve holistic care by linking care givers*. The expertise center Pharos had exerted a positive influence on standards of care in the Netherlands, as well as performing 'group advocacy' functions.

Lacking systematic evaluation studies, it was difficult to single out 'good practices' in the other categories. In the field of treatment, we focused on two methods which attempted to combine attention for physical, mental and social problems ('holistic care'). In the category 'prevention', we highlighted a program of creative and recreational activities for children in asylum centers.

4.1.3. Spain

(1) Traditionally, emigration from Spain has far outstripped immigration: even today, some two million Spaniards live abroad. Between 1850 and 1970 many Spanish migrants went to work in the growth economies of Northern Europe and Latin America. Immigration into Spain started to grow in the 1960's but remained at a low level until the 1980's and 1990's, when the economy expanded greatly. It increased from 198,042 in 1981 to 1,109,060 in 2001. In that year, immigrants made up 2.74% of the total population; the largest group (30%) came from the European Union, followed by Morocco and other African countries (27%), Latin America (26%), Asia (8%), and other European countries (7%).

Estimates of the number of undocumented migrants in Spain vary between 200,000 and 300,000, amounting to 18% - 27% of the total of registered foreigners. This is one of the highest figures in Europe. Spain has one of the lowest birth-rates in the world, with a virtually static population, and immigrants help to offset the economic effects of this situation.

Since the establishment of Spain's parliamentary monarchy in 1978, Spanish governments have implemented various policies to regulate immigration and further immigration. Several amnesties have been offered to undocumented migrants. Legislation introduced in 2000, however, had the effect of criminalizing and (further) marginalizing this group. As in Portugal (see below), attitudes to immigrants among the Spanish public are relatively tolerant. However, in the last few years they have become more negative and immigration has become a controversial political issue.

As far as asylum seekers are concerned, the rate of applications is very low (9,490 in 2001) the rate of rejections high (around 90%). While the application is being processed, asylum seekers are accommodated in centers run by the government or NGO's. The experiences of professionals working with asylum seekers and refugees suggests high levels of stress resulting from the flight itself and the living conditions on arrival. This applies even more to undocumented immigrants.

(2) Before the transition to democracy in 1978, Spain provided an example of the 'Southern European' welfare model, with the Catholic church providing many health, education and welfare services and a strong emphasis on family as care provider. Since the transition, however, care provisions have come increasingly to resemble those in the rest of Europe.

The Spanish health care system has been set up as an integrated National Health Service, which is publicly financed and provides nearly universal health care free of charge at the point of use. Service provisions are mostly publicly owned and managed, while governance of the system has recently been decentralized to all the regions. The general practitioner functions as gatekeeper to the rest of the health system. Social services are managed partly by the Ministry of Labor and Social Affairs, and partly by the Autonomous Communities who plan and regulate local services, co-ordinate resources and oversee their assessment and control. As yet, there is relatively little interest among professionals in issues concerning multicultural service provision, but some research has been undertaken on this topic.

Since 2000, foreigners living in Spain have the right to health care and social services, even if their situation is irregular. However, they have to undergo a registration procedure and obtain a special card in order to actually use the services. Fear, ignorance and administrative obstacles prevent some from obtaining this document.

(3) Asylum seekers and refugees form a very small part of the population and it is likely that many victims of political violence enter the country illegally. Asylum seekers are fully entitled to health and social care, and alongside the regular care system there are some specialized services provided by NGO's (religious or lay). Some of these services also offer help to irregular immigrants. These services tend to be concentrated in Madrid and Barcelona.

(4) The research carried out for the present study located several organizations offering (mental) health care to asylum seekers, refugees and migrants (including irregulars). A pioneer center in SAPPIR in Barcelona, which deals with many new arrivals. In the same city, SATMI is a privately financed body offered support to professionals working with these groups. EXIL is a program of medico-psycho-social rehabilitation for immigrant victims of human rights violations and torture. In Madrid, similar organizations were not found, but some initiatives are working in that direction, such as CASI (Social Care Centers for Immigrants). The Red Cross has established psychological assistance services for asylum seekers and refugees in March 2000, in different cities such as Madrid, Barcelona, Córdoba and Valencia.

Concerning professional education, although the attention to migrant problems in the regular courses is extremely scant, we located a fair number of initiatives in different sectors attempting to remedy this situation. Interest in these issues seems to be rapidly expanding.

Treatment methods used in the special centers mentioned above are very diverse. Preventive activities are organized by many NGO's working with migrants; they include legal advice, assistance in finding work, language and computer courses, and social or recreational activities.

4.1.4. Portugal

(1) In many respects the context of interventions in Portugal resembles that in Spain. Traditionally, Portugal has been a country of emigration, not immigration: in the 20th century, the main destinations were North America, Northern Europe and Brazil. As a nation, therefore, the Portuguese are very familiar with the phenomena of migration and ethnic diversity. Like all European colonial powers, Portugal experienced a wave of

immigration after the transition of its colonies to independence. This took place abruptly and chaotically in 1975, following the revolution in 1974 which ousted the dictator Salazar. Post-colonial migrants came from the PALOP (Portuguese speaking African) countries: Angola, Cape Verde, Guinea-Bissau, Mozambique, Saint Tome and Prince.

Towards the end of the 1990's, as in Spain, labor migrants begin to enter Portugal in larger numbers, mostly from Eastern European countries (especially the Ukraine). The work available was mainly in the construction and service industries. Immigration control is less strict than in Northern European countries, and amnesties have been offered to irregular immigrants in 1992, 1996 and 2001. The government has taken measures to combat discrimination and facilitate access to education and the labor market. As in Spain, however, the last few years have seen a tightening of immigration policy.

Concerning asylum seekers, Portugal operates an exceptionally restrictive policy, rejecting around 97% of applications. Only a few hundred asylum seekers are admitted annually. However, these figures conceal the fact that many victims of political violence probably enter the country as irregulars. Many probably also come from PALOP countries and fall in the category of 'post-colonial' migrants. Our research included interviews with asylum seekers and refugees in Portugal concerning their difficulties. Many reported problems of access to services, caused by bureaucratic obstacles and language difficulties.

(2) Like Spain, Portugal was formerly an example of the 'Southern European' welfare model, but since the 1974 revolution care provisions have followed the model of other European countries. Health care is covered by three overlapping systems: the National Health System (SNS), special insurance schemes for certain professions, and voluntary private health insurance schemes. Although the general practitioner is supposed to act as the gatekeeper to secondary care, in practice many people report directly to the emergency department in hospitals.

All aliens legally residing in Portugal have the same rights as nationals to use the National Health System. However, multicultural health care is not yet officially recognized as an issue, though there are sporadic signs of interest among professionals. We conducted an interview survey among service providers, which revealed that professionals often go to considerable efforts to find *ad hoc* solutions to the problems of helping immigrants, at the same time adhering strongly to the principle that all users should have access to the same kind of care.

(3) As we have seen, the category of asylum seekers and refugees is numerically very small in Portugal and hardly any special services of any kind exist for this group. These that do exist are mostly organized by the Portuguese Refugee Council (CPR). However, the emphasis in the activities of both the CPR and the Portuguese Government lies on matters more directly concerned with practical problems and integration (housing, training and employment). In these areas, we noted a relatively large number of interventions. Concerning health and social care for refugees, the one innovation which we managed to locate is described in the following section.

(4) This study found hardly any initiatives directed at improving mental health and social care provisions for refugees and asylum seekers. This has partly to do with the small numbers in these categories, but it also reflects the lack of attention to issues of cultural diversity in service provision generally.

The only initiative which might qualify for the category of 'good practices' is CAVITOP, the Portuguese Support Center for Victims of Torture in Portugal. CAVITOP is an NGO which forms part of the Coalition of Latin-European Centers for Victims of Torture (Latin-European CCVT). It was implemented in 2002 with the main goal of supporting and rehabilitating victims of torture, violence and cruel or inhumane treatment at a national level. However, the organization was not specifically set up for refugees.

Users are provided with a range of services (medical, psychiatric, psychological, social and juridical). In general, the first contact is made with a psychiatrist. After evaluation, the person is either assisted by CAVITOP, or referred to other NGO's or professionals. Since the organization was being set up at the time the present research was being carried out, we were unable to carry out any kind of appraisal of its activities.

4.2. Results of the Implementation Study

4.2.1. Transfer of 'Breathing Space' project from the UK to the Netherlands

The most suitable component of the Breathing Space project for transfer to the Netherlands was judged to be the 'Bi-Cultural Team': a low-threshold, culturally sensitive, 'one-stop' service for referring those in need to the appropriate mental health or social care agencies. After the Kent team had produced a manual describing the British project, a strategy for implementation in the Netherlands was worked out in a series of meetings by a team of experts drawn from Pharos and mental health service providers.

One important problem concerned the target group. The Breathing Space project was developed against the background of a large and fairly static concentration of asylum seekers and refugees in London. In the Netherlands, on the other hand, asylum applications, investigations and accommodation are located in different places, spread all over the country. The majority of asylum seekers are accommodated in centers and moved around the country at the behest of the government. However, in the Randstad (Rotterdam, The Hague, Amsterdam and Utrecht) some 10,000 – 20,000 asylum seekers live outside the centers, and for this group a service like the 'Bi-Cultural Team' would definitely be useful. The service would also be helpful for refugees with a residence permit who experience difficulties in accessing regular care provisions. At the same time, the project could also create opportunities for refugees to obtain work in the care sector, something which is otherwise extremely difficult to realize.

The scheme would in principle have to be paid for from the regular sources of health care financing. However, there were doubts as to whether it would be seen as an eligible form of service provision. A more suitable source of finance might be the public health budgets of local authority health services.

A special fund was located which could finance a small-scale pilot version of the project, but applications to this fund could only be made by mental health service providers. Unfortunately, none were interested in doing this. Because of strict new rules, numbers of asylum seekers were shrinking rapidly; they were expected to be halved within a year. Many facilities would be closed and the new policy was to keep all asylum seekers in accommodation centers. At the same time, service providers were being affected by a serious financial squeeze.

To sum up, the project was overtaken by rapid changes in the context for intervention – in particular, the sharp decline expected in the target group. Despite the disappointing outcome, valuable lessons were gained in this project about the complex considerations involved in transferring even the most promising interventions from one country to another.

4.2.2. Transfer of the Pharos school programs from the Netherlands to the UK

The Dutch research team prepared a manual on the schools program. Six different programs were described, three for refugee children in primary schools and three for those in secondary schools. Some programs could also be used for 'newcomers' in general.

After receiving this manual, the UK researchers met with representatives of schools in Britain which had indicated that they might be interested in implementation, in order to discuss a strategy for implementation. The most obvious problem concerned the differences between the British education system, in which refugees and children seeking asylum attend regular schools, and the Dutch system, in which they attend special schools. A second problem concerned financing: staff have to be trained and some programs even require two teachers for each session. Thirdly, there was no agency in Britain comparable to Pharos which might provide organizational support. In spite of all these practical problems, responses to the content and philosophy of the Pharos programs were extremely positive.

It was decided to proceed towards implementation at 'grassroots' level, involving initially one or two schools and education authorities, and then move towards wider implementation. The team felt was that the primary-school programs would be the easiest to implement. Finally, the need was recognized to involve refugees themselves in the running of the programs.

These problems were further discussed by the British team of experts and a joint meeting with Dutch experts was held in Brussels, at which participants from education authorities in Gloucester, Manchester and Kent agreed to take the program further in their localities. An e-mail discussion group was also set up. Subsequently, a delegation from Manchester visited the Netherlands to view the programs at first hand, and a Dutch team

The process of implementing the Pharos programs in the UK has made a very promising start. Following the meeting in Brussels, a delegation from Manchester visited the Netherlands to view the programs first hand and have been impressed with the results. This was followed up in 2004 by a visit of Dutch experts to Manchester, where plans to implement some of the Pharos programs are in an advanced stage.

5. DISCUSSION AND CONCLUSIONS

In this section we reflect on the lessons that have been learned from the study, as well as its implications for the development and transfer of good practices in the mental health and social care of refugees in Europe. One point should be emphasized at the outset: European policies concerning asylum and immigration are currently in a state of considerable turmoil. Realities 'on the ground' are continually changing and research may rapidly be overtaken by events.

5.1. Problems and opportunities presented by the study

This project was the first attempt to undertake a systematic comparative study of the mental health and social care of refugees in Europe. It called attention to a general lack of specific data on the mental health and social care of refugees, both at national level and at the level of individual service providers.

In each country, specialist NGO's and Refugee Councils played a vital role in terms of service provision for this group. However, the majority of refugees had to rely on 'mainstream' services for meeting their needs, and for this majority we can say that *care provisions for refugees and asylum seekers are only as good as those for migrants in general*. Our research indicated that in all countries, there was a shortage of education, training, monitoring and research relating to the specific needs of migrants in general, and refugees in particular. In the United Kingdom and the Netherlands, more attention had been paid to these issues than in Spain and Portugal. However, even in the former countries, problems concerning the accessibility and quality of services for migrants remain a source of concern.

5.2. The challenges faced by EU countries

5.2.1. Refugees and undocumented migrants

At the present time, many EU countries are reporting a dramatic decrease in asylum applications. This is seen as a consequence of tougher border controls, more rigorous screening of applications, swifter deportation and further restrictions in welfare support. However, as a consequence of these measures it is likely that people will continue to enter EU countries but be less inclined to seek asylum when they arrive, thus swelling the numbers of undocumented migrants. It is important therefore to examine the lessons from the Southern European countries in the provision of health and social care to undocumented or 'irregular' migrants.

5.2.2. Avenues of Access

There were important differences in the pathways through which refugees enter countries and the impact this may have on the provision of mental health and social care services. This can be appropriately referred to as the avenues of access through which refugees receive services, and these have been identified as an important area for comparative study. The countries studied drew attention to at least three avenues of access.

- The UK operated largely a dispersal system in which asylum seekers were given social support on condition that they agreed to be dispersed to areas outside of the south east of England. Areas of dispersal were often ill prepared to receive asylum seekers and the early stages of dispersal were often fraught with problems. However, in some areas gradually innovative approaches to service delivery emerged, typically in a 'bottom up' fashion.

- In the Netherlands, most asylum seekers were more closely controlled within Accommodation Centers, where specialized medical teams provided intake and referral to regular mental health and social care services. The approach here is more uniform and systematic than in the UK, but is also, arguably, less innovative and dynamic. Since the mid-nineties, the Dutch government has actively discouraged the setting up of categorical facilities for refugees and asylum seekers, on the grounds that adequate services must be provided in the regular care system.

- In Spain and Portugal the situation is again different. A significant majority of migrants enter the country clandestinely and consequently are not entitled to immediate access to health, mental health or social care. Undocumented migrants only have access to the emergency services of public hospitals. Both users and service providers may be extremely badly informed about each other.

5.2.3. Barriers to access

The *right* to care is one thing; good *access* to care may be quite another. Usually, access to services is via professional gatekeepers. Barriers may arise from the gatekeepers' lack of knowledge and cultural competence in dealing with refugee clients. This may be compounded by the refugees' own lack of knowledge of the health care system. 'Brokers', 'advocates' or 'mediators' thus have an important role to play in ensuring good access and appropriate referral.

5.3. Recommendations for the Development of Minimum Standards

Our findings led us to conclude that, in broad terms, good practice in the mental health and social care services for refugees includes the following components: *cultural sensitivity*, an *integrated approach, political awareness* and *accessibility*. Those services that have been identified as offering good practice have combined, to a greater or lesser degree, these four components. In the main report (Waters and Ingleby, 2003), we have elaborated this argument further.

A landmark European Council Directive dated 27 January 2003 has laid down minimum standards for the reception of asylum seekers. As a complement to these guidelines, we would suggest the following guidelines for the provision of mental health and social care services to asylum seekers and refugees:

- An assessment of mental health needs is undertaken at an early stage of the asylum seekers application;
- The assessment is sensitive to the particular culture and language of asylum seekers and includes interpreters and translated materials where required;
- Advocacy services are available to help meet the range of mental health and social care needs asylum seekers and refugees may have;
- Key service providers, including those acting as gatekeepers, receive training modules to develop their skills and awareness in dealing appropriately with this client group;

- Asylum seekers and refugees are consulted about the sort of services they would find helpful;
- Mental health and social care services are responsive to the stages of the asylum process and provide support at key phases during which clients may be most vulnerable.

Our research has shown that there are complex local variations in the context of care provision, which lead to widely divergent solutions, but that exchange of ideas and practices can still be of great value. Those working in this field can gain new insight into their own situation by comparing it with that of others. The authors sincerely hope that this report marks the beginning of an extensive program of development in this field.

6. ACKNOWLEDGEMENTS

The authors gratefully acknowledge the support of the European Refugee Fund, which provided 80% of the financing for this project.

Thanks are also due to the following agencies which collaborated in the project:

- *United Kingdom:* Home Office, Department of Health, Department for Education and Skills, Refugee Council, and Medical Foundation for the Care of Victims of Torture.

- *The Netherlands:* Pharos Refugee and Health Knowledge Center; ALTRECHT (mental health care conglomerate for the Utrecht region); GGZ-NL (organization of Dutch mental health service providers).

- *Spain:* University of Barcelona, SAPPIR (Servicio de Atención Psycho-patológica y Psicosocial a los Immigrantes y Refugiados), in particular Joseba Achtegeui.

- *Portugal:* Open University, Lisbon (CEMRI - Centro de Estudos das Migrações e das Relações Interculturais), in particular Natália Ramos and Lígia Ferreira; Portuguese Refugee Council (Conselho Português para os Refugiados), in particular Mónica Farinha.

REFERENCES

Gijswijt-Hofstra, M. and Porter, R. (eds.) (1996) *Cultures of psychiatry and mental health care in postwar Britain and the Netherlands*. Amsterdam: Rodopi.

Ingleby, D. and Watters, C. (2002) Refugee children at school: good practices in mental health and social care. *Education and Health 40*, 43-45. Available in pdf format at http://www.sheu.org.uk/pubs/eh.htm .

Kleinman, A. (1981) Patients and healers in the context of culture: an exploration of the borderland between anthropology, medicine and psychiatry. Berkeley, CA: University of California Press.

UNHCR (2003) Asylum applications lodged in industrialized countries: Levels and trends, 2000-2002. Geneva: United Nations High Commissioner for Refugees (www.unhcr.ch) .

Watters, C. (2001) Emerging paradigms in the mental health care of refugees. *Social Science and Medicine 52*, 1709-1718.

Watters, C. (2001) *Evaluation Report on the Breathing Space Project - an innovative mental health project for refugees and asylum seekers*. Canterbury: University of Kent.

Watters, C., Ingleby, D., Bernal, M., De Freitas, C., De Ruuk, N., Van Leeuwen, M. & Venkatesan, S. (2003) *Good practice in mental health and social care for asylum seekers and refugees*. Final Report of project for the European Commission (European Refugee Fund). Canterbury: University of Kent. Copies of the report are available at cost price from the second project leader, e-mail J.D.Ingleby@fss.uu.nl, address: ERCOMER, Utrecht University, P.O. Box 80.140, 3508 TC Utrecht, The Netherlands. The report can also be downloaded in Word format at www.ercomer.org/staff/DIN.html .

AUTHOR INDEX

SUBJECT INDEX

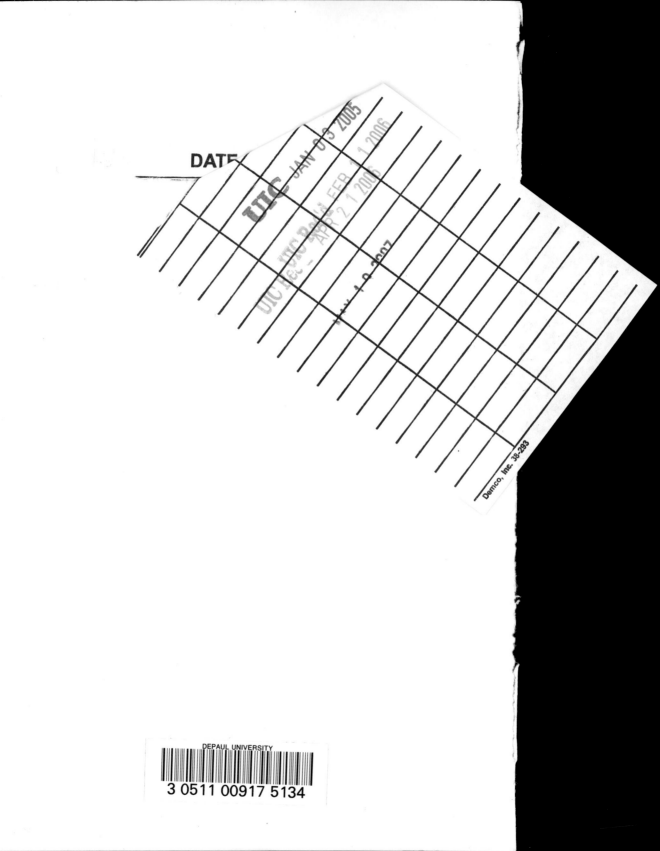